THE SOCIAL NETWORK DIET

Change Yourself, Change the World

Miriam E. Nelson, PhD
and
Jennifer Ackerman

Published by FastPencil PREMIERE

Published by FastPencil, Inc.
3131 Bascom Ave.
Suite 150
Campbell CA 95008 USA
(408) 540-7571
(408) 540-7572 (Fax)
info@fastpencil.com
http://www.fastpencil.com

White Bean and Escarole Soup on page 77 used with permission from Eating Well, Inc. (eatingwell.com). Wheatberries with Fruit and Honey-Orange Dressing on page 81 from Strong Women Eat Well by Miriam E. Nelson and Judy Knipe, copyright © 2001. Used by permission of G.P. Putnam's Sons, a division of Penguin Group (USA) Inc.

Cover graphic design by Dan Seward.

Back cover authors' photograph by Elinor Ackerman.

First Edition

"Hats off to Dr. Nelson for illuminating the critical but often overlooked ways that social networks can contribute to our health. And for giving us very clear maps for building the supportive communities we need to create vibrant health every day."

Christiane Northrup, MD, ob/gyn physician and author of the New York Times bestsellers: *Women's Bodies, Women's Wisdom* and *The Wisdom of Menopause*

"The Social Network Diet is a strong, smart, one-of-a-kind guide to making healthy change in your own life and in the lives of those around you. Social revolutions start with an individual and ripple from person to person, city to city, across the country. If social networking can change governments, why can't it change how we eat and manage our weight? Well, it can. In this game-changing book, Dr. Miriam Nelson tells you how your simple human interactions can make you—and those around you—successful in being fit and healthy once and for all."

**Nancy L. Snyderman, MD, FACS,
NBC News Chief Medical Editor**

"The Social Network Diet offers a powerful combination: highly effective advice on diet and exercise…and innovative strategies for improving our communities."

**Michael F. Jacobson, PhD, Executive Director,
Center for Science in the Public Interest**

"The Social Network Diet explores an essential ingredient for enhancing health: people coming together to support one another. As CEO of a leading global health service company, I have seen firsthand the power of social networks."

David M. Cordani, President and CEO, CIGNA Corporation

Also written by Miriam E. Nelson, PhD

(with Sarah Wernick, PhD)
Strong Women Stay Young
Strong Women Stay Slim
Strong Women, Strong Bones

(with Judy Knipe)
Strong Women Eat Well

And Kristen R. Baker, PhD, and Ronenn Roubenoff, MD, MHS
(with Lawrence Lindner, MA)
Strong Women and Men Beat Arthritis

The Strong Women's Journal

And Alice Lichtenstein, DSc
(with Lawrence Lindner, MA)
Strong Women, Healthy Hearts

(with Lawrence Lindner, MA)
Strong Women, Strong Backs

And Jennifer Ackerman
The Strong Women's Guide to Total Health

Also written by Jennifer Ackerman
Notes from the Shore
Chance in the House of Fate: A Natural History of Heredity
Sex Sleep Eat Drink Dream: A Day in the Life of Your Body
Ah-Choo! The Uncommon Life of Your Common Cold

To Eliza, Alexandra, Zoë, and Nell

❧

Contents

Introduction

This book will help you make healthy changes in your life by improving your environment—and in so doing, transforming the world. It is not your classic diet book. It is not an exercise manual. It is unlike any other nutrition and physical activity plan you have ever seen. It is a guide, rooted in exciting new research, on how to make lasting, positive change in your life by creating a supportive social network and a favorable food and physical activity environment.

There is so much misinformation in the media these days, especially when it comes to nutrition and exercise. People are smart and want to make meaningful change in their lives through credible guidance supported by real evidence. This book offers just that—evidence-based counsel brought to life by personal stories of success and proven strategies for achieving your goals.

The first step is to understand the nature of the problem. We're facing an overwhelming epidemic of poor nutrition, inactivity, and excess body weight in this country. More than two-thirds of Americans are overweight or obese. And even for those who aren't overweight, it's still difficult to eat as well as one would like and exercise as much as one needs to stave off weight gain.

For decades we've been told that our creeping overweight and lack of physical activity is our fault—that we lack self-discipline, that we're lazy, that we're self-indulgent. With such an accusatory finger pointed at us, it's no wonder we despair.

But is our overweight and unhealthy lifestyle really our own fault? Do we simply lack willpower? Are we just lazy over-eaters?

I don't think so.

Take Martha Peterson At the age of 51, Martha's weight had ballooned to a high of 210 pounds. She was living in Atlanta at the time, a city with serious obstacles to healthy living—among them, roads made for driving, not walking, and a tradition of heavy southern cooking. Many of Martha's Atlanta friends were also overweight. "I had pretty much given up on exercising," she says. Then, in 2009, Martha moved to Denver. There she found an environment more conducive to physical activity and good nutrition, as well as a network of friends with an active, healthy lifestyle. A little over a year later, she had lost 53 pounds, was walking regularly with her new friends, joining a neighbor for spinning classes at the local recreation center, and eating better than she ever had.

As Martha's story suggests, our food intake and physical activity are not matters of simple willpower. New research backs this up. Study after study suggests that the crisis we're facing as individuals and as a nation is only minimally caused by our own poor choices—it is primarily a reflection of our surroundings, both our social and our physical environments. Complicated forces have converged over the past several decades to create an overall environment toxic to healthy eating and activity. Our family upbringing, the communities in which we live and work, large cultural shifts, economic factors, and local and national policies have all fostered the development of this unhealthy environment. We're surrounded by unhealthy food—and messages to eat that food—and by barriers that keep us from being physically active. Whether we live on the East or West Coast or somewhere in between, in an urban, suburban, or rural area, we face huge obstacles to healthy living.

In other words, it's not just you; it's the company you keep and your surroundings.

Only recently have we become aware of how tight the relationship is between people and their environment. This concept, known as the socioecological model, recognizes that our behavior is shaped to a large extent by forces outside of our control, in our social and physical surroundings. A slew of factors beyond willpower affect our health and health-related behavior, from our genes to our family dynamics, social ties, and the place we live.

Habits are hard to change. But when your environment changes, so do your habits. The point is this: To make healthy living easier, we need to create an environment that supports our health rather than sabotaging it. Fortunately, we now have the tools to do so—key among them, social networks.

When we hear the term "social network" these days, we tend to think of online networks. But social networks are as old as humankind itself. They are defined simply as groups of people and the connections between them. Social networks are complex, powerful entities that shape our thoughts and habits and can function either to our detriment or to our advantage. There is even emerging evidence that behavior within social networks is contagious, spreading from person to person. For years, we've known that social networks influence who smokes, who drinks, who contracts sexually transmitted diseases, even people's happiness. Now we understand that they can also have a profound influence—either positive or negative—on our body weight and physical activity levels.

Consider this: Studies show that people are far more likely to become obese when a close friend becomes obese. This has proven true not just for adults, but also for teenagers. This "peer weight" impact is particularly powerful among women—and also overweight adolescents. Moreover, when you look at weight issues among large groups, even whole nations, the really powerful large-scale impact of social networks emerges: People are most comfortable weighing slightly less than the norm in their social networks. But if that norm creeps upward, they find higher and higher weights perfectly acceptable. In other words, as weights deemed acceptable rise, the new, higher norm spreads from person to person.

On the other hand, social networks can also have a beneficial effect on weight control. One 2008 study showed that if a spouse loses weight, the partner loses weight as well. There's equally strong evidence that people are more effective at losing weight when they embark on weight loss programs with friends. In one study, people were recruited to participate in a weight loss program—some with friends to support their weight loss efforts and some without such a "friends network". Those with the friends network (whether they were old friends or newly acquired friends) were much more successful at losing weight and maintaining healthy behaviors over the long term.

Right now it takes a real effort to make healthy choices, even for those of us who are motivated and have a supportive social network. Despite our best efforts, less than a third of American women maintain a healthy body weight. We try to eat well, but the average person gets 35 percent of her calories (750 calories

per day) from added sugars and unhealthy saturated fats—
that's 23 teaspoons of added sugars and three and a half tablespoons of solid fat. And we aren't dishing these teaspoons of
sugar out of the sugar bowl or digging into the Crisco can.
This sugar and fat is embedded in our food. Our food supply
has seen dramatic shifts in the past thirty years or so, with
more and more foods available to us that are cheap, convenient, and mostly unhealthy. We have also witnessed dramatic
changes in *how* we eat—we cook less, eat fewer family meals
and consume more meals while watching television, working
at our desks, or riding in our cars. In addition, we move less
throughout the day.

Not all of us can change our lives by moving from one location to another, as Martha did. Nevertheless, we can do a lot to
alter our social and physical environments. Restructuring your
personal environment takes focus, time, and effort, but it's
well worth it. You'll see from the strategies offered in this book
that just shifting one or two elements in your environment can
make a big difference. And seeing how effective these simple
changes can be gives you the confidence—and the tools—to
make additional, more ambitious changes. One success leads
to another. Moreover, when you alter your own surroundings
—even if the shift is subtle—it has a ripple effect, changing the
lives of those around you, your family, friends, and community.

It's my belief that creating change on a large scale begins
with personal action.

This book grows out of new research conducted with my
colleagues at Tufts University looking at what makes for successful life change, both within individuals and within society.
We have analyzed pioneering movements such as one to pre-

vent childhood obesity and another to reduce heart disease risk in midlife women. Most recently, we studied the strategies of women across the country who have successfully improved the nutrition and physical activity environments in their own communities and beyond. I consider these women "game changers." They offer inspiration and practical guidance on harnessing social networks to generate lasting positive change in their own lives and in the world at large.

Women, it seems, are powerful catalysts—in large part because of their effective use of social networks. One woman, Deanne, tackles her own obesity by altering her personal environment and then urges others like her toward similar lifeshifts. Neelam brings gardens and fresh produce to inner-city Los Angeles and unites with likeminded community members to oust sugar-sweetened beverages from schools. Barbara joins with citizens and city planners to create the concept of "complete streets" to foster walking and biking to work. Jill recruits young high school graduates to help improve recess and active play in schools around the country. And Carla develops a program in Maine to get children and their families moving in the winter, a program that has been adopted by most northern states. Throughout the book, but especially in the final two chapters, you will read about and learn from these and other game-changing women.

There's a *New Yorker* cartoon I've always loved. It shows a pack of wolves howling in unison at the moon. One wolf leans over and says to another: "My question is, are we having any impact?" Though people in my field have been working hard to get out the message and move people toward healthier habits, the mountain of physical inactivity and poor nutrition is bigger than ever. We need to make change *now* in this arena and in many others—hence the urgent call for each of us to become engaged in this effort.

Given how much is at stake and the scope of the challenges facing us, our generation understands that we can't sit back and wait for things to change. We need to support one another. We're already influencing the people around us. Now we need to do so in a more deliberate way, to spread positive change quickly. This is the beauty of social networks. They can help us do together what we cannot do alone. Not only can they support our own personal lifestyle changes, but they also are essential for creating large-scale change. We need to mobilize our collective energy to improve our own lives and the lives of our families, communities, and beyond. This is what it will take to create the big change we need in this country. Together, we can create an environment that promotes good health for one and for all.

Chapter 1. It's a Complicated Web

When I give my talks to the public, I often show a series of maps of the U.S., year by year, from 1985 to the present. The effect is always shocking. The maps show each state in a color that indicates obesity rates—from cool, blue colors for low obesity to warm, fiery colors for high obesity. Over the 25 years, the overall color of the map gradually turns from light blue to darker blue to pale red to darker red, to bright orange. By 2009, most of the country is either red or orange, indicating that more than 30 percent of the population is obese. It looks like the spread of some horrible epidemic. And it is. What the map doesn't show is that another 35 percent of our population is overweight.

Not long ago, my husband came to one of my talks. As we were driving home, he said, "Mim, you've been working in the field of nutrition for a long time, overlapping almost identically with the obesity maps you showed. I know you've been working hard, but what have you been working on? It's a good question and one I've thought a lot about over the past five years. When I think of the billions of dollars that have gone into research, public health, and education since the mid-1980s, I have to ask, "Have we been focusing our efforts on the wrong target?" For years, we've emphasized individual responsibility. We need to refocus our lens in light of new research showing that these approaches don't work if an individual's social and physical environment remains unchanged.

Obesity Trends in U.S. between 1985 and 2009

1985
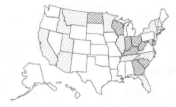

1986
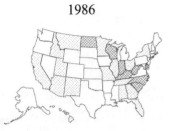

1987
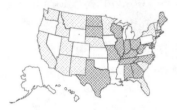

1988
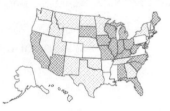

1989
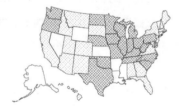

1990
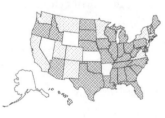

1991
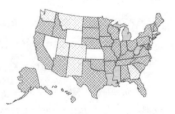

1992
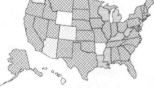

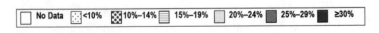

No Data   <10%   10%–14%   15%–19%   20%–24%   25%–29%   ≥30%

1993
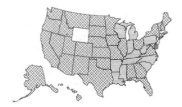

1994
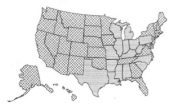

1995
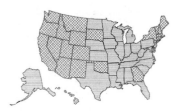

1996
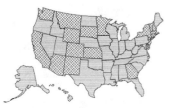

1997
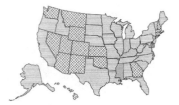

1998
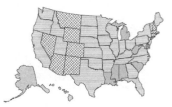

1999
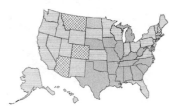

2000
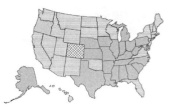

No Data | <10% | 10%–14% | 15%–19% | 20%–24% | 25%–29% | ≥30%

2001
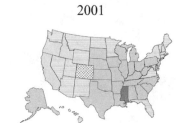

2002
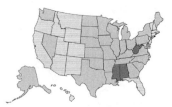

2003
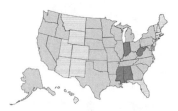

2004
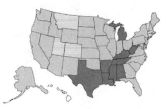

2005
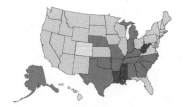

2006
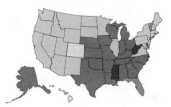

2007

2008

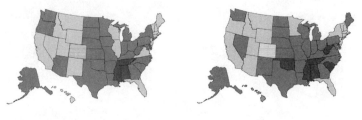

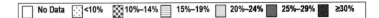

No Data ⬚ <10% ⬚ 10%–14% ⬚ 15%–19% ⬚ 20%–24% ⬚ 25%–29% ⬛ ≥30%

2009

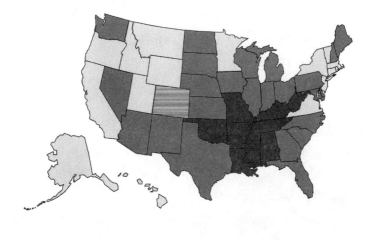

| No Data | <10% | 10%–14% | 15%–19% | 20%–24% | 25%–29% | ≥30% |

Every year since 1985, the Centers for Disease Control and Prevention has tracked obesity rates for every state. (Obesity is defined as a body mass index over 30 and/or roughly thirty pounds overweight.) The darkening colors indicate higher obesity rates. Southern states have the highest obesity rates, but every state now has very high rates. The state with the lowest obesity rate is Colorado.

THE SOCIAL NETWORK EFFECT

Over the past few years, innovative work suggests the surprising power of our environment in shaping our lives. Especially fascinating is research showing that our social environment—the network of people we spend time with, our family, friends, and peers—has a profound influence on our health and our health-related behaviors.

In 2007, researchers Nicholas Christakis and James Fowler of Harvard Medical School released a study that sent shock waves through the public health community. The study looked at 12,067 people tracked over more than three decades and found that the risk of becoming obese spread almost like a virus from person to person. Analyzing data from the Framingham Heart Study from 1971 to 2003, the researchers used sophisticated statistical modeling to examine whether weight gain in one person was associated with weight gain in his or her friends, siblings, spouse, or neighbors. Their findings: In married couples, if one member became obese over time, the likelihood of the other following suit increased by 37 percent. Among siblings, if a woman became obese, her sister's risk rose by 40 percent.

Most astounding, however, was the impact of friends—even friends living far apart. In fact, the researchers suggested that friends have an even greater effect on people's risk of gaining weight than their genes do. A person's chance of becoming obese appeared to climb by 57 percent if a friend of the same sex became obese. (There was no effect found for neighbors or for friends of the opposite sex.)

It gets even more interesting. The closeness of the friendship matters. Among close mutual friends, if one friend became obese, the other friend's chances of doing so increased by 171 percent.

Three additional studies support this "contagion" theory of obesity. A 2008 study reported results of an analysis of adolescents. In a school-based survey of 90,000 youth in grades 7 through 12, students were asked to list as many as 10 of their closest friends (5 male and 5 female). The study showed that an adolescent's body weight correlated strongly with his or her friends' body weights. The impact was strongest in girls and in adolescents with higher body weight.

Another 2008 study looking at 1,000 people in each of 29 nations in Europe also supports the theory that weight gain ripples through peer networks. The study revealed that people's body weight tended to reflect the weight of those around them. The highest body mass index (BMI) for men, it turned out, is in Malta, Slovenia, and Greece; the lowest in Turkey, the Netherlands and Italy. For women, the highest is in Malta and the lowest, in France and Italy. But in all countries body weight has been increasing.

The most recent study was published in December of 2010. Intrigued by the Harvard study, Dr. Rena Wing and colleagues at Brown University decided to test the hypothesis on a younger group of people, ages 18 to 25. They surveyed 288 young men and women in Rhode Island. The results showed that overweight and obese men and women were more likely to have romantic partners, best friends, and casual friends who were also overweight. (They also observed that overweight and obese men and women with more social contacts trying to lose weight had a greater intention of losing weight themselves. If a friend is trying to lose weight, this seems to influence a young adult's own desire to lose weight.)

Why is there such a powerful "friend" effect? Our current theory is that when someone becomes obese, it makes it more socially acceptable for people close to that person to gain weight. The change in social norm of acceptable body size can spread quickly, rippling through networks like rings spreading from a pebble thrown into a pond, even among people who live hundreds of miles away from one another. The spreading effect is more pronounced in friends of the same gender. Gains in weight appear to spread through a population—with friends and relatives apparently influencing other friends and relatives, for example—in a way reminiscent of a contagious disease.

The point is this: We choose the weight at which we're comfortable, bearing in mind the weights of our peers. This is because we care about our status and position in society. If we assume that relative slimness confers status, it makes sense that we would choose to weigh a little below the norm in our social networks. But as that norm creeps up, we're comfortable having our own weight creep up, too—as long as it remains close to the weight of our peers. When my friends get a little fatter, I feel okay about becoming a little fatter myself. As a scientist in this field, I believe that these changing norms have had a profound influence on the rapid spread of obesity.

Eating is a social activity

When it comes to social influences, it's not just norms that affect us. Who we eat with matters, too. So does the way we were raised. Deanne Hobba's experience is a good example of this. Deanne had been heavy all of her life. Most of her family members and friends were heavy and inactive. She grew up in a huge Italian family where everything revolved around food, she says: "Every Sunday, we had these giant pasta meals, and the refrain was always 'eat, eat, eat.' Every family celebration centered on food. I grew up thinking that's the way it should be, and it was very hard to break out of this mindset."

Eating is a highly social activity, and perhaps not surprisingly, we model our habits on those of the people around us, especially family. What your parents ate while you were watching them across the table affects what you eat now. (However, contrary to popular belief, their admonitions to eat your fruits and vegetables did not result in greater consumption of same! Parental influence appears to be much stronger if parents model good eating habits, consuming plenty of fresh fruits and vegetables rather than just talking about how one should eat them.)

Cultural influences in families can also affect what you eat. Studies of Hispanic adults in this country show that those who are less acculturated to American habits and stick more to their traditional customs consume more fruit, rice and beans, and whole milk, whereas those who are more acculturated eat more fast food, snacks, sugar, sugar-sweetened beverages, and foods with added fats. One small study that compared the eating habits and feeding practices of French and American parents found an interesting twist: In the U.S., parents more often use food as a reward or to regulate a child's emotions than do parents in France.

But by far the most significant parental influence on eating habits is the family meal. Family dinners are a foundation of healthy food choices. Children who eat dinner with their families every day eat more fruits, vegetables, and whole grains and more calcium- and iron-rich foods. They also drink less soda and eat less fried food and fewer saturated fats and transfats. Moreover, studies show that teens who eat more than three family meals a week are less likely to skip breakfast and more likely to eat fewer fast-food meals. The effect is lasting. One study revealed that young teens who eat regular family meals in middle school have better quality diets and eating patterns five years later when they're in high school.

As for the influence of spouses and significant others: We tend to eat what they eat. This makes sense, of course. Once people become involved in a relationship, they often shop, cook, and eat together, typically merging their food choices, especially at dinner. One study showed that dietary changes for women followed a pattern, with women in a heterosexual relationship eating meat more often and drinking higher-fat milk than they would if they were alone.

Our food choices are also affected by our dining companions outside of family. When researchers looked at the way adolescents choose items from a typical lunch menu, they found that the students admitted that their peers' choice swayed their own choices. Most often they opted for soda, chicken, hamburgers or cheeseburgers, and fries. However, they did try to balance their unhealthy lunches with healthier, more nutritious family dinners. (More proof that family dinners matter!)

And here's a twist for women: As it turns out, we consume more calories if our dining companions are also women. Researchers who studied students at three large university cafeterias in Ontario, Canada, found that women were more likely to choose foods with higher calories when they were eating with members of the same sex. On average, women who ate with other women consumed 665 calories during their meal; when they dined in groups of four women, their intake jumped to an average of 800 calories. But women who ate with a lone male companion consumed only about 550 calories and —in a reversal of the "more the merrier" trend with all-women groups—those who ate with a group of men took in fewer calories, only 450.

The point is, social networks are powerful forces in shaping our ideas about our health and also, our health-related behaviors. But it's not as simple as that. While social influences are strong, genes and environment also have supporting roles.

Deanne's story points out just how complicated the interactions can be between genes, environment, and social influences. She had tried many times to trim down, she says—to watch what she ate and to exercise regularly. But she always fell back into her old habits, being inactive, eating large portions at meals and snacking on junk food, cookies, chips, candies. At age 33, she weighed 268 pounds and suffered from high blood pressure, high cholesterol, and frequent migraine headaches. That year, 1999, two things happened.

"It was the summer, and I had taken my nephew to the amusement park," Deanne recalls. "On one ride, they kept trying to bring the bar down over me, and then it would spring back up. The staff asked me to get off the ride because the bar wouldn't close. I was so embarrassed. I knew I had to do something, but still I put it off. That winter, I was working in a hospital, and I helped move people who were too heavy to get about themselves, and I thought to myself, 'I could be looking at myself in 20 years' time—unless I do something now.'"

These events triggered some astonishing changes in Deanne's life. But how did she become one of those 35 percent of women in the U.S. who are obese? The answer lies in the socioecological model, the complex interplay between the individual, our relationships, our community, and societal factors.

Socioecological Model

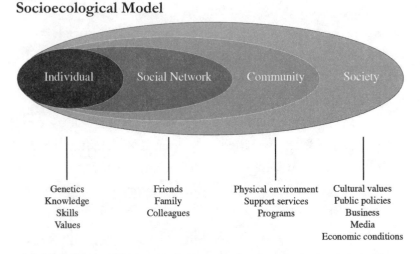

Multiple factors influence our behaviors related to physical activity and nutrition. Our genes, personal beliefs, and values; our social network; our food physical environment (the foods that are in our house, at work, and in our community: public transportation, sidewalks, parks, and community resources for physical activity); larger cultural norms, and industry, business, and government policies all influence what we eat and how active we are.

YOU, THE INDIVIDUAL

Beyond your social networks, what personal issues affect how much you eat and your level of physical activity?

Genes, for certain. We've known for some time that body weight is a matter of balance between food intake and energy output. Among the intriguing new insights we have learned lately is that this balance is controlled not by conscious will-power, but by a powerful, unconscious biological system. A significant piece of this system is genes, which influence everything from taste preferences and appetite to how much fat we burn.

To date, scientists have identified 198 genes that are related to body weight. We all possess these genes. They affect our tendency to eat sugary, fatty foods, to store fat (rather than burn it), and whether or not we want to run around or prefer to spend time on the couch. They are potent forces, and we've had them in place in our DNA for more than 10,000 years. They evolved when we were hunter-gatherers facing scarce seasonal food supplies, to promote eating and reinforce its pleasures and to conserve fat and reduce energy expenditure.

If you think about it, having the capacity to lay on fat and conserve it makes sense from an evolutionary standpoint, especially for women. For thousands of years, having a little extra weight helped us remain fertile and deliver a healthy child. Now, even when food is readily available and easy to obtain, we have the same genes that we had when food was scarce and hard to come by, and our bodies still crave calories and defend overweight with a vengeance. That's why it's so hard to take off the pounds—and even harder to keep them off.

We're just beginning to understand how specific genes contribute to differences in body weight—the ways in which variations in these genes can have a profound effect on everything from how we metabolize food to how much energy we expend with physical activity—as well as how these genes operate in families. Deanne knew she was struggling against her own genetic legacy: She came from a background in which overweight was prevalent on both sides of the family.

But there's another side to the story. Genes do not act in a vacuum; they're heavily influenced by their immediate environment. Fascinating insights have come from a new field called epigenetics, which explores how environmental factors can affect the behavior of our genes.

In a nutshell: Genes need instructions on what to do and when to do it. They are a little like the keys on a piano. There they sit until the player presses them to make a sound. The player is something called our "epigenome" (meaning in addition to, or above, the genome), which contains chemical switches that instruct genes, helping them decide when to "express" themselves, to switch on or off. As it turns out, diet, exercise, stress, and other factors can activate these switches. Moreover, the responses that are triggered can be passed along through generations.

Consider this surprising theory. Conditions in your mother's womb may affect your epigenome, and hence, the way your genes behave throughout life. This is known as the Fetal Origins Hypothesis. A pregnant mother's diet can influence her child's epigenome, for instance. Some foods (e.g., sesame and sunflower seeds, shellfish, spinach, broccoli, and peppers) contain compounds that become part of the epigenome or affect it, determining the way genes act not just in utero, but into adulthood. Similarly, a pregnant mother's unhealthy weight gain and obesity during pregnancy can turn on specific existing genes that influence the future body weight of her children. Studies suggest that a child born to an overweight mother is three times more likely to be overweight by age 7 than a child born to a normal weight mother, and may also face a lifelong risk of type 2 diabetes.

Oddly enough, the reverse is true, too. Malnutrition and underweight can have a similar effect. In fact, the first inkling that a mother's diet and body weight could influence her baby's genes in utero came from studies of the offspring of parents who suffered through the Dutch famine during World War II.

It's an intriguing story. In late 1944 and early 1945, parts of the Netherlands suffered severe famine; rations for adults ranged from only 400 to 800 calories a day. Mothers were sorely undernourished, as were their unborn babies. Studies revealed that babies conceived or born during this famine period were predisposed to early heart disease, type 2 diabetes, and obesity. It was as if evolution had devised a mechanism to make offspring conceived or gestated in a time of deprivation more able to conserve energy.

If we perturb the system either way, it seems, our genes automatically go into a kind of default mode toward conserving energy. So if your mother was either underweight or overweight during pregnancy, you may be predisposed to being overweight throughout life.

Our genes also drive our food preferences, what we like to eat. Studies of the dietary habits of twins suggest that genes influence our preference for certain types of foods, including shellfish, flour and grain products, rice, vegetables, fruit, and dairy products. In fact, genetic variance explains between 30 and 50 percent of our leaning toward certain kinds of foods. Tim D. Spector of the Twin Research and Genetic Epidemiology Unit at King's College, London, where many of these twin studies have been conducted, suggests that much of our preference for foods is set before we are born. "More often than not, our genetic make-up influences our dietary patterns," he says. One study of Danish and Finnish twins in 2010 found that even our preference for white or rye bread is influenced by genetic predisposition.

Our physical activity levels, too, may be determined in part by genetic variations. One recent study at the University of California, Riverside, found that the drive for daily exercise is a trait that may be passed along genetically to successive generations—at least in mice. The experimenters found that they could selectively breed mice to produce offspring that were "high runners"—that is, they had increased levels of daily activity to about three times the normal level. The female mice raised their levels by running faster; males boosted it by spending more time running. The researchers speculate that this may help us find ways for women and men to more easily step up their activity. Perhaps women would find it easier to boost their workouts by doing more intense exercise, and men, by increasing the duration of their exercise.

In the human domain, evidence from twin studies suggests that genes could be involved in our inclination to be sedentary or physically active. One large study compared identical and fraternal twins, ages 19 to 40 years, from six European countries and Australia. The subjects were classified as "physically active" if they reported at least one hour of exercise each week. It turned out that differences in exercise behavior were about 60 percent attributable to genes. Scientists suggest that a number of genes probably affect this propensity to be physically active or inactive. Right now, they're poorly understood, but their influence is strong.

YOUR SURROUNDINGS

While our social network and genes play a powerful role in our health, it's not only who our parents are and the company we keep that makes it hard for us to eat well and stay fit. Our larger environment also plays a part, from our food supply to our physical surroundings.

When Neelam Sharma moved to South Central Los Angeles with her two young children in 1996, she discovered a dismaying problem: "I wasn't really able to access what I thought was good, affordable, high-quality food." South Central L.A. is a low-income area with a population of about 1.36 million. Neelam observed that residents in her community had little or no access to fresh fruits and vegetables and other healthy foods. There was no supermarket within walking distance. "I really resented having to drive so far to get basic food items," she says. She had grown up in England and recalled working in the family garden with her father. "I remember growing berries and spinach; some basic items we used for Indian cooking were always grown in the backyard." The lack of access to healthy food in her new neighborhood shocked her.

South Central L.A., like other low-income areas in this country, has been what some experts call a "food desert"—a densely populated community with a scarcity of supermarkets but an abundance of convenience stores and fast-food restaurants. In these areas, residents may have to travel miles to reach a well stocked, full-service grocery store where fresh produce and other high-quality, healthy food is readily available at lower prices. (Convenience stores have prices that can be as much as 76 percent higher than those found at grocery stores and they rarely carry fresh produce.)

Easy access to supermarkets is linked with healthier eating. For example, a study of African Americans found that those who lived in neighborhoods with full-service grocery stores ate more fruits and vegetables than those in neighborhoods without these stores. On the flip side: The absence of fresh-food markets in neighborhoods is linked with higher body mass index, especially for low-income Americans. So too is a high density of fast-food restaurants and convenience stores. These "food desert" neighborhoods often have high rates of obesity and diet-related diseases.

The problems in South Central L.A. are not unique. They're emblematic of the challenges that face us all over this country: Our food supply—fast, cheap, convenient, but often unhealthy —makes it hard for us to eat well and creates what many of us call a "toxic" food environment. These toxic environments can be in urban, suburban, or rural areas.

American Idle

Much of the focus on our struggles with weight has centered on food intake. But lately, researchers have begun to look at other factors affecting the weight-gain equation: our low levels of physical activity, for instance. If our food environment makes it hard for us to eat well, maybe there's something about our physical environment that makes it hard for us to get sufficient physical activity.

Whether or not we're active is certainly determined in part by personal factors: our own propensity for exercise, for instance, and our willingness to make time for it. Genes affect how exercise makes us feel; social networks can exert pressure for or against regular exercise. We're learning now that our physical surroundings may also influence whether we lead active lives: Our jobs, homes, even the design of our communities can either encourage or hinder physical activity as a part of daily life.

When Barbara McCann was a journalist working in Atlanta in the 1990s, she wanted to ride her bicycle to the office. The city, however, was "not a very good place to do that," she recalls. Like Martha Peterson, she found Atlanta an environment somewhat hostile to healthy living. Streets had no bike lanes and there was little interest in creating them, which made biking hazardous and unpleasant. "The way the city approached transportation was extremely traditional, very automobile oriented," says Barbara. Unfortunately, Barbara's experience in Atlanta is all too common. Many of our communities have been engineered in ways that discourage biking, walking, and other kinds of routine physical activities.

The Physical Guidelines for Americans recommends getting 150 minutes of moderate intensity activity or 75 minutes of vigorous activity over the week to maintain health. Almost all Americans fall short of this goal. Children are the most active, but still only 10 percent or less meet the guidelines. With each decade of age, the percentage diminishes. Most active are highly educated people, as well as those who live in western states such as Washington, Colorado, and Oregon; least active are those who reside in southern states such as Kentucky, Louisiana, and Mississippi. A quarter of Americans report being completely inactive during their leisure time.

These statistics are distressing, but they're not new. Levels of reported exercise haven't changed much in decades. What's different now is that we're getting less physical activity in the course of our daily routines. We're not moving as much in our jobs, in taking care of our homes, in commuting or running errands, or just going from place to place. An example of the decline in daily movement was revealed in a poll not long ago in which seven in ten Americans said they walked or rode a bike to school when they were children. Today, only one in ten school-aged children do so.

SHIFT HAPPENS

There's no question that environmental factors play a part in inhibiting healthy eating and active living in this country. Our food supply produces cheap calories in great abundance—at steep cost to our waistlines and our health. Our jobs, our new technologies, our ways of commuting, even the design of our communities have "engineered" natural daily movement out of our lives, making it harder to stay fit.

Until we can create change in the larger environment, for the moment, it falls to individuals to make the personal change they need to transform their lives, just as Martha and Deanne did.

When Deanne made her life transition, she started small. To revise her "horrible" eating habits, she joined Weight Watchers, which helped her structure her eating and taught her not just what to eat but how to eat. "When people ask me how I did this," she says, "I tell them that I started with small steps and was incredibly persistent. When I first decided I was ready to lose weight I was huge, 125 pounds overweight. I told myself, 'Well, I have to start somewhere—I'll just try to lose a little weight, any amount.'"

Deanne began by changing what she put into her personal environment. She examined the portion sizes she was eating. "They were so distorted," she recalls. "They were based on what I had grown up with. Whatever was put in front of me, I ate.

"I started to measure out my food. I prepared portions ahead of time—e.g., chicken cut into 6-ounce portions. When I made meals, I pulled out only what I needed to eat for a single portion for a single meal, so there was no temptation to go back for seconds.

"That first week, I lost four pounds, and I realized I didn't have to starve myself to death. I could do this. That small success really fueled itself. When I was drawn to food, I learned to ask myself, 'Are you hungry?' More often than not, the answer was, 'No, just bored.' So I would just turn away from the food instead of eating, waiting for the wave of 'hunger' to pass." She began a regular program of walking on a treadmill, building up to a half-hour a day. She bought my first book, *Strong Women Stay Young*, and began lifting—at first with cans of beans and later with real weights. From February to November of 2000, she lost 60 pounds. Then she joined a gym and began jogging on the treadmill and exercising on an elliptical. She also found a new social circle. "I still maintain my old friendships," she says, "but now I have a whole new group of friends; we train together and run races together." Just five years later, by age 39, she had lost 120 pounds.

These days, Deanne weighs 145 pounds and wears a size 8. More important, each week she runs 25 miles and bikes 75 to 100 miles; she swims three times a week and can dead-lift more than 100 pounds. She races in triathalons and marathons. Still, even after all of these years, Deanne admits that she has to make conscious decisions every single day to eat well and go to the gym. "I just take it day by day," she says. "I ask myself: Am I going to the gym today? Am I going to eat properly? Am I going to consume that doughnut or bagel sitting on the office counter, which I don't need because I just ate a healthy breakfast a half hour ago? When I make a mistake, I never beat myself up. If I eat badly at one meal, I don't batter myself and say, 'Well, there goes the day.' I try to get back on track as soon as I can."

Deanne has maintained her weight for more than eleven years. She says that she has never been happier.

You see now that a complicated web of forces in your environment shapes what you eat and how you move. But what forces have shaped the environment? Before we can make the change we want to see in ourselves and in our world, we need to understand how our environment came to be what it is today.

Chapter 2. Living Large

As long ago as 1949, the late nutrition scientist Ancel Keys speculated that our social and economic circumstances might produce an epidemic of obesity. He predicted that overeating and expending less energy would become an issue, leading to problems with weight control. "While our calorie intake goes up our output goes down," he wrote. "The wonderful advances of technology do not merely free us from back-breaking toil; they make it almost impossible to get a decent amount of calorie-using exercise."

Keys was right. Over the past half century or so, potent forces have molded our food supply and our built surroundings, creating an environment that sabotages our efforts at healthful eating and physical activity. How? What is going on here?

My research at Tufts University and my work on two government committees offer some answers. In 2008, I was asked to be a member of the Dietary Guidelines Advisory Committee to help the government develop the 2010 Dietary Guidelines for Americans. For two years, I joined twelve other leading nutrition scientists in delving into the newest science on nutrition and health. This was an incredible experience. It was also challenging. This committee has a long tradition of taking conservative, politicized positions on the question of the American diet. The challenge for me was to try to move it in a new direction. Fueled by concern about the current obesity epidemic, I was particularly interested in understanding what Americans actually eat. What do they eat too much of and too little of? How has this changed over the past four decades or so? There's no denying that what we consume has changed. What does the overall food environment look like? How is what we eat now different from what we used to eat? What about where we eat and where we purchase foods? Finally, I wanted to understand better how we got to this place of unhealthy eating. Very few Americans eat well. Why? And why is the modern American food supply such a catastrophe?

WHAT DO WE EAT?

We eat more. We're eating more than we did forty years ago, at least in terms of calories. In the 1970s, young women ate just over 1,600 calories a day; in 2000, consumption jumped to more than 2,000 calories a day. Similarly, midlife women went from 1,510 calories to 1,828 calories, and older women went from 1,325 to 1,596 calories. Most of these extra calories come in the form of added sugars, unhealthy added fats, and refined grains. (The good news is that calorie intake from 2000 to 2008 has remained relatively stable.)

The top five foods sources for calories in the American diet are:

1. Grain-based desserts and snacks (cakes, cookies, dough-nuts, pies, crisps, scones, muffins, cobblers, and granola bars)
2. Yeast breads (especially refined white flour breads)
3. Chicken and chicken mixed dishes
4. Soda, energy drinks, and sports drinks

5. Pizza

Grain-based foods in the 1970s added 432 calories per day to our diets; now they contribute an average of 625 calories per day. Similarly, added fats contributed 403 calories per day in 1970 and now add 616 calories per day. Calories from vegetables and fruits have remained steady at approximately 125 and 80 calories per day, respectively.

Lots of SoFAS. The biggest contributors to the increase in calories in our diet come from solid fats and added sugars (known as SoFAS). Solid fats are unhealthy fats such as saturated fat and transfats. Added sugars come from an ever-expanding variety of sources such as high fructose corn syrup and sucrose. These ingredients add calories to food but offer minimal nutritional value. Consumption of these solid fats has risen from 56 pounds per person per year in 1970 to 87 pounds per person in 2008. Added sugars have jumped 15 percent from 119 pounds per person in 1970 to 136 pounds in 2008.

Excessive sugar of any kind appears to affect blood levels of hormones involved in appetite and eating, including insulin, leptin, and ghrelin, and may play a role in the development of diabetes and obesity.

The recommended number of calories from SoFAS should be between 5 and 15 percent of total caloric intake. But today, the average American, young or old, male or female, gets 35 percent or more of their calories from SoFAS. The typical woman 40 years of age is consuming 758 calories a day in SoFAS—from 3.5 tablespoons of solid fat and 23 teaspoons of added sugars per day. One in ten American women is consuming more than 1,000 calories a day in SoFAS, and only 5 percent of women are getting 300 calories a day or less from them.

Where are these calorie-boosting SoFAS coming from?

The top five contributors to added sugars in our food supply are:

1. Sugar-sweetened soda
2. Grain-based desserts and snacks
3. Fruit drinks
4. Dairy-based desserts
5. Candy

The top five contributors to unhealthy solid fats are:

1. Grain-based desserts and snacks
2. Regular cheese
3. Sausage, franks, bacon, and ribs
4. Pizza
5. Fried potatoes (French fries and hash browns)

More refined grains. Refined grains are a big culprit contributing to excess caloric intake. I want to be very clear: We're not talking about whole grains here. It's smart to eat whole grains in abundance, because these grains are digested slowly, satisfy hunger for longer periods of time, and provide fiber and other nutrients. However, of the 7.5 ounces of grains consumed per person per day in this country, less than 1 ounce is whole grains. The rest are refined grains, which have a lower fiber content than whole grains and are largely devoid of nutritional value, with the exception of some important vitamins. They also have lower concentrations of the minerals, essential fatty acids, and phytochemicals that are vital to health.

Not all refined grains are equally guilty. For example, plain pasta and white rice are not major contributors to daily caloric intake. But refined grains that act as a vehicle for added sugars and unhealthy fats add huge numbers of calories to our diet. In fact, as you have seen, the single biggest food group that swells our calorie intake is refined grains—cookies, cakes, other dessert foods, and snacks. These grain-based foods are also the top contributor to our intake of solid fats and the number two contributor to added sugars. The past few decades have seen a sharp increase in our intake of these foods. Between 1970 and 2005, total per capita availability of refined grains rose by 41 percent.

More sodium. We also consume too much sodium. Excessive salt contributes to chronic disease, especially hypertension. Sodium intake in the American diet has risen steadily in the past few decades. Now the average American gets 3,436 mg of sodium per day—more than twice what is recommended by the 2010 Dietary Guidelines. Some 5 to 10 percent of this occurs naturally in the foods we eat. Another 10 percent arrives with our use of the salt shaker. This means that the lion's share of our salt intake—75 to 80 percent—comes from processed foods. The leading contributors to excessive salt consumption include yeast breads, chicken and chicken mixed dishes, pizza, pasta and pasta dishes, lunch meats (cold cuts), condiments, and sausage, franks, and bacon.

Dietary Intakes Compared to Recommended Goals or Limits

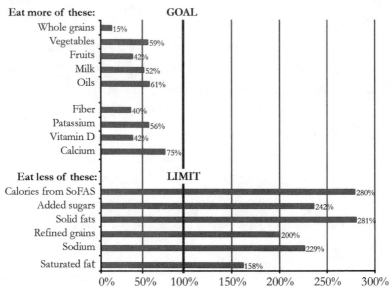

Unfortunately, the average American's diet contains far too few healthy foods and nutrients and far too many foods that provide empty calories and other unhealthy ingredients. Bars show average intakes for all individuals (ages 1-2 years or older) as a percentage of the recommended goal or recommended limit.

(Source: What We Eat in America, National Health and Nutrition Examination Survey 2001-2004 or 2005-2006)

Less milk and more sweet drinks. In general, we drink less milk than we did three decades ago and more sweetened drinks. Our intake of beverage milk dropped 33 percent from 1970 to 2008. Meanwhile, we started drinking more sodas and more fruit drinks, including fruit juice cocktails and ades, such as sports drinks. By 2008, our stores carried twice as much fruit drink (almost 13 gallons per person) as fruit juice (almost

7 gallons per person) and more than twice as much carbonated soft drink (almost 47 gallons per person) as beverage milk (around 21 gallons per person). The availability of carbonated soft drinks jumped 20 percent, from 39 gallons per person in 1984 to 47 gallons per person in 2008. That works out to roughly 250 12-ounce cans per year for each person. Now we also have a huge increase in fruit drinks, sports drinks, sweetened coffees, smoothies, iced tea, ades, and other sweetened beverages. In a single year, the average American drinks about 60 gallons of these sweet drinks, at a cost of $500 per person and an addition of some 85,000 calories.

The calories contained in beverages vary widely, from 50 calories to 250 calories in an 8-ounce serving. For teenagers and young adults, sugar-sweetened beverages, especially sodas, are the leading contributor to calories. Sodas and fruit drinks tend to add calories to our diet without providing nutrients. Fat-free or low-fat milk and 100 percent fruit juice may contain an equal number of calories, but they offer abundant nutrients as well. Sugar-sweetened sodas also contribute 36 percent of the total added sugars to the American diet. (If we simply removed these sodas from our food supply, Americans would be a lot better off. More about this in Chapter 3.)

Water and coffee and tea provide fluid for hydration with no calories, unless, of course, one loads them with sugar.

More cheese and meat. We eat close to four times as much cheese today as we did a half century ago, up from about 7.5 pounds per person per year to almost 30 pounds. This is almost entirely the result of eating more packaged and prepared foods containing cheese and cheese products, such as pizza, bagel spreads, burritos, nachos, and fast-food sandwiches. The average American also eats almost 200 pounds of meat, poultry, and fish each year—an increase of 50 pounds per person from a half-century ago. While our consumption of beef, pork, and lamb has remained stable over the past couple of decades, we're eating a lot more chicken. We should be eating more fish.

More fruits and vegetables. In the good news department, per capita fruit and vegetable availability is up 19 percent since the 1970s. But we still don't eat enough of these healthy foods. The average fruit and vegetable consumption for women is just under two servings of vegetables and one serving of fruit per day, about half the recommended amounts. Also, we tend not to seek variety. Much of the rise in consumption of fruits is limited to apples, bananas, and grapes—and a good share of it is in the form of highly processed snacks. The rise in vegetable consumption is primarily limited to tomatoes, onions, and leafy lettuces. Potatoes still dominate our vegetable intake and orange juice, our fruit consumption. Although I count a good old-fashioned baked potato as a vegetable, the majority of potatoes we eat these days come in the form of fries or chips or as part of a processed meal. And unfortunately, some 80 percent of total tomato consumption comes from processed tomato products such as sauces, canned tomatoes, tomato paste, and ketchup.

WHAT HAS CHANGED IN THE WAY WE EAT?

Almost as dramatic as these changes in *what* we eat are changes in the *way* we eat. Fifty years ago, most of us ate family meals sitting down at a table, with no TV in sight. Now we eat on the run, at fast-food counters, in our cars, at our desks, and in front of our computers or the television. For many Americans, it's a rare occasion to eat at the dinner table with family and friends. As mentioned earlier, the percentage of families who eat a meal together each night across the country has dropped by 20 percent over the past three decades. Studies show that families who do not dine together do not eat as healthily, consuming more fried foods and soda than families who share meals.

Our new way of eating includes:

Bigger portions. Over the past few decades, portion sizes have ballooned, with the largest increases in hamburgers, French fries, soda, and baked goods. A hamburger is now 112 percent bigger than it used to be. Bagels are three times larger; muffins, four times. Portions of food and beverages served in restaurants and fast-food places are often at least twice as large as the standard serving size defined by U.S. Dietary Guidelines. The average serving of steak is 224 percent larger than established standards, and a chocolate cookie, 700 percent larger. The original Burger King meal of burger, fries, and soft drink contained about 600 calories. Today's supersize portion of the same meal holds more than 1,500 calories. A standard soda fountain drink used to be 7 ounces; now it's 12 to 42 ounces. At movie theaters and other soda fountain venues, cups have expanded to 32 or even 64 ounces. The bigger the container, the more soda we're likely to drink. This is also true of food: the bigger the plate or bowl, the more we eat. And unfortunately, the size of our dinnerware has grown in the last few decades, with the average plate two inches larger in diameter than it used to be.

Eating on the run. With our jam-packed schedules, too many of us forgo leisurely, mindful meals at a table in favor of eating haphazardly while we're on the go, in our cars or at our desks as we finish that project or make that important phone call. A 2005 survey found that 20 percent of restaurant meals were purchased at drive-through or curbside venues, up from 14 percent in 1998. (I'm on a personal mission to get companies to do away with drive-throughs—as you can see, I haven't been very successful.) A 2006 survey by Nationwide Mutual Insurance found that almost half of young Americans and a third of baby boomers say they eat full meals in the car and an even larger number of snacks there.

"Screen time," especially television-viewing. Some two-thirds of Americans have the television on during dinner. Studies show that food intake increases when we watch TV because distraction impairs the brain's ability to perceive and monitor the amount of food we're consuming. In one study, subjects asked to eat macaroni and cheese while they watched TV lost all track of how much pasta they were consuming and ate more than those who were focusing only on their food. Moreover, whenever we watch TV, we are showered with food-related advertisements, which affect our appetites and our intake. Especially vulnerable are children and adolescents. Research shows that more than half of TV ads viewed by young people promote snacks and sweets, fast foods, and sugar-sweetened beverages. These ads have been found to encourage children to request high-calorie, low-nutrient foods and beverages.

More foods away from home. From 1970 to 2008, the share of an average household budget's disposable income spent on foods eaten away from home rose 26 percent, while expenditures for foods eaten at home dropped 42 percent. Even more dramatic is the jump in our daily caloric intake from foods eaten outside the home. In 1977, it was about 18 percent; over the next couple of decades, it expanded to 77 percent. We also devote less time to food preparation these days. We used to spend 90 minutes a day preparing food; now it's closer to 50 minutes. We used to eat out at restaurants and fast-food places only about twice a week; today, it's more like once a day. This is partly because more women are working outside the home and have busier lives, with longer commutes. Also, many families have dual incomes, so there's more money to spend eating out. To meet demand, the number of commercial eateries has increased 89 percent, while the number of cheap, convenient fast-food restaurants has risen by 147 percent. In many places in this country, there are 24-hour fast-food eateries on nearly every corner.

Unfortunately, when we eat at restaurants or fast-food places, we tend to consume more calories because portions are larger and there are few healthy foods. A typical restaurant meal has about 1,000 to 2,000 calories. Also, what we eat is generally a lot less healthy than what we serve at home. Recent research from the USDA found that when we eat meals outside the home, we boost our daily intake of calories, fats, alcohol, sodium, and added sugars, and we reduce our vegetable consumption. A 2005 survey found that women's top three most popular foods ordered in restaurants or for takeout were French fries, hamburgers, and pizza, often loaded with excess added fat, salt, and calories.

The changes in our diet noted above have resulted in part from dramatic shifts in our food supply.

Shifts in the Food Environment Since the 1970s

Food Environment Measure	Time Frame	Percent Change
Number of commercial eating places	1972 to 1995	89%
Number of fast-food restaurants	1972 to 1995	147%
Percentage of meals and snacks eaten at restaurants (non-fast food)	1977 to 1995	150%
Percentage of meals and snacks eaten at fast-food restaurants	1977 to 1995	200%
Food "at home" expenditures by families and individuals as a share of disposable income (% of income)	1970 to 2008	-42%
Food "away from home" expenditures by families and individuals as a share of disposable income (% of income)	1970 to 2008	-26%
Total food expenditures by families and individuals as a share of disposable income (% of income)	1970 to 2008	-24%
Share of daily caloric intake from food away from home	1977-78 to 1994-96	77%
Average number of items carried in a supermarket	1978 to 2008	449%

(Source: 2010 Dietary Guidelines Advisory Committee Report, USDA, USHHS)

HOW HAS OUR FOOD SUPPLY CHANGED?

Food is cheaper. Americans use less of their incomes for food than do people in any other developed country in the world—just 11 percent, compared with 22 percent in Europe. The American food system has surrounded us with food choices based largely on convenience and cost. Fifty years ago, our selection was limited to what was produced by small local farms. Now most of our food comes from supermarkets supplied by large agribusinesses in other states or countries. A typical American farm, for instance, once raised a flock of a hundred or so free-ranging chickens; now a commercial broiler growing house raises some 20,000 chickens. Policies at the national level have driven this change. Modern industrial agriculture, subsidized by taxes, has forced many small farmers out of business.

This modern system has made food less expensive. It has also expanded our food choices. In the 1950s, the average grocery store had about 2,000 food items for sale; in 1978, it was just over 10,000. Now most carry some 45,000 to 70,000 food items. Every year, another 17,000 food items are introduced to grocery store shelves. Nearly all of these are convenient, cheap, and highly palatable. This would seem to be a good thing except for one important fact: Much of this food is not wholesome.

Most foods now packing our grocery-store shelves are highly processed, containing little food value and too much sugar, fat, and salt to be considered healthy. Food companies understand that these ingredients are cheap, irresistible to our taste buds, and highly rewarding to the pleasure pathways in our brains, so they design their products with this in mind. They also market them heavily. According to the USDA, food manufacturers spend $12 billion a year advertising their highly processed, highly packaged products; only 2 percent of this advertising is devoted to fresh fruits and vegetables, and beans and grains.

Where we eat our food and buy our food has also shifted, away from smaller grocery stores and toward warehouse clubs and supercenters that offer food packaged in bulk sizes.

Food Expenditures as Percentage of Disposable Income

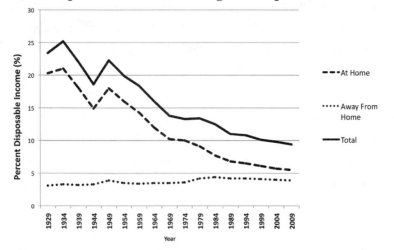

Since 1929, the average American's expenditure on food as a percentage of disposable income has dropped. The largest drop in spending has been on foods eaten at home. The U.S. population spends less on food than do people in any other developed nation.

(Source: USDA Economic Research Service)

Past agricultural policies have failed us. We are producing, processing, purchasing—and ultimately eating—far more corn and grain than we need and not enough fruits and vegetables. It's interesting to note that this country does not currently produce sufficient fruits, vegetables, and whole grains for its citizens to consume the amounts recommended by the U.S. Dietary Guidelines. We need 7.4 million more domestic acres of land in production to provide enough fruits and vegetables and whole grains for Americans to meet the guidelines. Yet we devote roughly five times more acres to corn and refined grain production than we need to fulfill our dietary needs. (Much of it goes into animal feed and fuel production.)

Moreover, a good share of what we produce contains a number of chemicals. Almost all non-organic farmers use pesticides on their crops. On a per/acre basis, the highest levels of pesticides are applied to fruit and vegetable crops. In livestock production, feed additives are used to speed the growth of animals, including antibiotics, tranquilizers, hormones, and arsenicals (drugs containing the poison arsenic). Not only do the animals that are raised this way carry chemical residues, but their accelerated growth results in a higher proportion of fat. For example, conventionally raised beef has 30 percent fat as opposed to 5 percent in a free-range animal; some 98 percent of this fat is of the saturated type known to contribute to heart disease in humans. The huge quantities of poultry, beef, pork, and other foods produced by these agribusinesses pass through a small number of hubs, where they're processed and distributed for transportation via road, rail, or water. The average food item travels more than 1,500 miles from farm to plate. An even more important issue is that these large agribusinesses block access to markets for smaller farmers.

On the positive side, we now have more fruits and vegetables available to us year round. But many of them are grown for easy transport at the cost of nutritional value and flavor. (We all know how tasteless a commercial tomato can be!) To prepare foods for a long journey, most products undergo some kind of processing. This helps to keep them fresh during their travels and sometimes, to make them look and taste better.

While limited processing is important to make foods safe, excessive processing almost always introduces unhealthy food additives. Nearly all processed foods contain several of the more than 10,000 additives used by major food companies to enhance texture, flavor, and color and to preserve and stabilize foods.

Among the most common ingredients in the processed foods on our supermarket shelves is high-fructose corn syrup (HFCS). This corn sweetener, a refined sugar with no essential nutrients, has found its way into nearly every nook and cranny in the larder, into everything from soft drinks and fruit drinks to flavored yogurts, cereals, jams, jellies, peanut butter, tomato sauce, ketchup, and baked goods. Thirty-five years ago, only 1 percent of sweeteners consisted of HFCS; now it's 42 percent. The average American takes in about 10 teaspoons of HFCS every day, equivalent to about 160 calories; and one in five people consume more than twice that amount.

It's worth pausing for a moment here to look at the story behind the key ingredient in this ubiquitous syrup—corn—because of the huge impact it has had on our food supply. What's behind this bloom of corn sweeteners?

While the U.S. government has assisted farmers with important conservation measures in the past five decades, it has also encouraged farmers to grow as much corn as possible, with the help of federal subsidies. Food companies have lobbied hard for this: When corn is plentiful, it is an amazingly cheap raw material for use in industry. Not only does it quickly fatten sheep, pigs, farmed fish, and especially cattle (at some cost to our health), but it also can be milled and refined to create ingredients in dozens of edible (though not particularly nutritious) products, from hydrogenated oil to hot dogs, bologna, frozen yogurt, and salad dressings—indeed, many of the foods that contribute to our excessive calorie intake.

Sugar, too, has enjoyed special protection in our country. As early as 1789, the First Congress of the United States imposed a tariff on foreign sugar coming into this country from the Caribbean to raise revenue. Eventually, the tariff had the effect of protecting the newly established sugar industry in Louisiana. Beginning in 1934, a series of "sugar acts" protected sugar producers, millers, and refiners from operating losses. Many of the protections are still in place, and the sugar industry contributes heavily to political candidates to preserve these protections.

In short, with the help of government subsidies, crops such as corn and sugar have become cheaper, and food companies have found innumerable creative ways to jam them into small, tasty, high-calorie packages that we have a hard time not gobbling up.

Fortunately, there is some good news on this front. The current administration has begun to reverse past policies to reduce those subsidies that have created this problem. Subsidies are now a minor incentive for producing sugar and HFCS. But the practice is so entrenched that it is going to take time to turn it around.

WHAT HAS SHAPED OUR PHYSICAL ACTIVITY ENVIRONMENT?

In the past half-century or so, a number of factors have conspired to make us expend less energy throughout the day. In the home, labor-saving devices from bread makers to vacuum cleaners have lessened the need for active household tasks like kneading and sweeping. In the early 1960s, 50 percent of jobs in this country demanded moderate physical activity. In 2011, that figure dropped to just 20 percent. This shift means that in a work day, Americans burn an average of 100 fewer calories than they did 50 years ago. Moreover, major technological innovations have reduced the number of jobs that require high-activity manual work from 30 percent to 22 percent. At the same time, low-activity jobs have jumped from 23 percent to 41 percent. The number of people employed in these jobs went from 16 million in 1950 to 33.7 million in 1970 and more than 58 million in 2000. Today, twice as many people work in low-activity jobs than in high-activity jobs. Most of us sit all day long.

Amounts of leisure time devoted to exercise have not changed much over the past half century. However, we now spend many more of these leisure hours than we used to at sedentary activities such as watching TV or using the computer, which expend little or no energy. I was amazed to learn that there are more televisions in the average American household (2.73) than there are people (2.55) and that half of American homes have three or more televisions. After work and sleep, TV viewing is the most time-consuming activity in this country, with the average American watching more than 4.5 hours of TV each day. (A television is on in the average American household for 7 hours and 40 minutes!)

But perhaps the biggest culprit contributing to our inactive living is the rise of automobiles for personal travel. Estimates show that in the U.S., there are 1.9 personal vehicles per household. The mean number of drivers in each household is 1.8. The average U.S. household, then, has more cars than drivers, and some 20 percent of households have three cars or more.

Trends in the Amount of Total Physical Activity

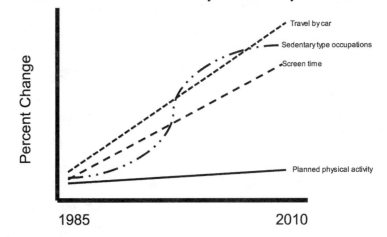

Adapted from RC Brownson et al, 2005

Over the past several decades, our pattern of physical activity has changed dramatically. While planned, intentional physical activity has remained the same or increased slightly since 1985, other lifestyle factors have made us more sedentary. Travel by car has increased and more occupations are sedentary. Moreover, Americans spend much more time in front of a screen (television, computer, tablet, smartphone, etc.). All of these factors contribute to a more sedentary everyday life for most Americans.

The car has become indispensable for commuting, shopping, and socializing, in large part because the "Freeway Era" from 1945 to the present has made our communities more sprawling. Studies show that when neighborhoods have a mix of shops and close-packed residences, as well as a grid of well-connected streets with sidewalks, people tend to drive less and walk and cycle more. Unfortunately, the past fifty years have seen a trend away from this kind of community design toward spread-out, automobile-dependent communities girdled by high-speed roads. In these environments, the private car is by far the safest, most convenient way to get to schools, neighborhood shopping, and public transportation stops. When polls ask Americans why they do not walk more, the answer is that the distance to stores, restaurants, and schools make them more apt to take the car. More than half say there are too few shops or restaurants within walking distance of their homes.

It's interesting to compare our experience in this respect with that of Europeans. Europe's cities are far more compact than our own, and people living there make one in three of their daily trips by foot or bicycle. In this country, it's one in ten. It's perhaps no coincidence that in several European countries, the obesity rates are a third to a half what they are in the U.S. (although many European countries are quickly catching up to us).

Over the past several decades, our surroundings—our food supply and physical activity environment—have become toxic to our health. Frankly, I'm surprised that more people aren't angry about this. Fortunately, awareness is growing. Americans are coming to understand that the trouble they're in results not from a failure of personal willpower but from an unhealthy environment—one that demands a lot of effort to eat well and be physically active.

The ultimate goal is to fix this larger environment. The first step in this direction is reshaping your own personal environment to support your health, just as Martha and Deanne did. If enough of us do this, the effect will ripple out, spread to others, and set us up for making the critical large-scale change this country so desperately needs. To get started, you need a strategy for understanding your own personal environment and the challenges it presents.

Chapter 3. Booting Up

"We are the environment, there is no distinction."
-David Suzuki, scientist and environmental activist

So the problem is clear: Our environment makes it difficult for us to eat well and be active. But how does one go about fixing that? How do you create an environment where living a healthy life is easier—where it requires less effort to eat well and move more throughout the day?

The first step is understanding what makes a healthy personal environment and then examining your own environment to see what needs changing. This chapter offers you the tools to do this—a picture of what you should be shooting for and a strategy for assessing your own situation.

One obvious way to change your personal environment is to put yourself in a radical new setting.

I love to climb mountains. When I attempt difficult ascents, I always have a qualified mountain guide with me. Over the years, my regular guide, Isabelle Santoire, has become one of my best friends and colleagues. For years, we have talked about how we would like to conduct a study in which we take women who want to lose weight and get in shape on a trip to high-altitude mountains—say, the Alps of France—for a week or two. The social environment would be extremely supportive. The women would be surrounded by friends, all aiming for the same goal. In the Alps, food choices are limited to what is available in the mountain huts. Getting to the huts requires physical activity in the form of hiking, and the altitude itself dampens appetite. No doubt everyone in the study would lose weight and become more fit. In fact, we've seen this very transformation again and again in women we've taken into the mountains.

Conversely, if Isabelle and I were to take a group to an all-inclusive resort in the Caribbean, where you can eat all you want and your choice is whether to stroll down to the beach to sunbathe or go work out at the fitness center, most women would likely gain weight. I'm not frowning on a trip to the Caribbean; I'm just suggesting that your environment either supports or hinders your ability to make healthy choices.

To bring this closer to home: Where you live in the United States influences your energy balance. Deanne notes that she grew up in a small, economically depressed coal-mining town in western Pennsylvania where there was no culture of exercise or healthy eating. Now she lives in a town north of Boston, Massachusetts, a town that promotes a healthy lifestyle, where she can easily walk to grocery stores, and where people run and bike in the big open spaces around the town. "If I'm out for even ten minutes, I see ten or more people out exercising. There was not much of that in the town I grew up in."

As Martha's story suggests, if you live in the South, you'll have a more difficult time maintaining fitness and healthy body weight, and if you live in Colorado or the Northeast or Northwest, it will be easier. (This is because the food environment and physical activity participation vary in different parts of the country, as do social networks and norms.)

The point is, it's important to understand the context in which you live and its profound influence on your health.

While most people can't just pull up stakes and move to a healthier place as Martha did, we can each reconstruct our own personal environment to make it easier to be healthy. We can do this little by little, in relatively easy ways, by removing one teaspoon of added sugars, one serving of refined grain, and one tablespoon of unhealthy fat at a time, and by building more physical activity into our lives, one step at a time.

WHAT SHOULD YOU STRIVE FOR?

Before you attempt to change your personal environment, it's wise to understand your targets for nutrition and physical activity.

From 2007 through 2010, I had the good fortune to serve on two federal advisory committees at the invitation of the U.S. Departments of Health and Human Services and Agriculture. The first was the 2008 inaugural Physical Activity Guidelines Advisory Committee, which I vice-chaired. The second, as I mentioned in Chapter 2, was the 2010 Dietary Guidelines for Americans Advisory Committee. Both of these committees delved into the latest research on nutrition and exercise so that our recommendations could draw on the best up-to-date evidence. What we learned was eye-opening, especially concerning how few Americans actually meet the current guidelines.

What is healthy eating?

The 2010 Dietary Guidelines committee report included some 660 pages reviewing the latest research, along with our recommendations; too big a bite for most people. I and a few other members of a forward-thinking subcommittee felt strongly that we needed to distill these findings to make them useful to the public. So we decided to boil down the report to just a few integrated recommendations that would have the greatest impact on health. We came up with four recommendations (more details at www.dietaryguidelines.gov): Three are related to nutrition and one, to physical activity.

The three nutrition guidelines can be summarized as follows:

1) **Eat a little less**. Consume smaller portions, especially of high-calorie foods; choose whole, minimally processed foods, especially when eating foods away from home.

Americans need to pay attention to their energy balance. People at different life stages—pregnant women, children, adolescents, adults, and older adults—have different energy needs. If you are overweight or obese, you need to focus on reducing overall calorie intake while increasing physical activity.

It is not easy to know your calorie needs, as a number of factors enter into the equation, including your body size, age, gender, level of activity, and even how much you fidget. The table below provides an estimate of energy needs for women who are at an ideal body weight. (Women who are heavier may have higher energy needs than those indicated here. Similarly, women who are lighter in weight may need less.) Ask yourself, "Am I maintaining my weight?" If so, then you are in energy balance. If you're gaining weight slowly over time, then you're consuming more calories than you're expending and may need to cut back. If you're losing weight, then your calorie needs are not meeting your total energy expenditure, and you may have to increase your intake. Use the table below only as a rough guide, as your needs may differ.

Estimate of Calorie Needs of Adult Women

Estimated energy needs in calories per day for ideal body weight women by age and activity level	Female/ Sedentary	Female/ Moderately Active	Female/ Active
Age	Calories		
19-20	2000	2200	2400
21-25	2000	2200	2400
26-30	1800	2000	2400
31-35	1800	2000	2200
36-40	1800	2000	2200
41-45	1800	2000	2200
46-50	1800	2000	2200
51-55	1600	1800	2200
56-60	1600	1800	2200
61-65	1600	1800	2000
66-70	1600	1800	2000
71-75	1600	1800	2000
76 and up	1600	1800	2000

(Source: 2010 Dietary Guidelines Advisory Committee Report, USDA, USHHS)

I also encourage you to know the calorie content of the foods that you eat, especially foods that come in packages or are served to you away from home.

2) **Shift your eating toward more plant-based foods,** especially vegetables, cooked dry beans and peas, fruits, whole grains, nuts, and seeds. Also, eat more seafood and fat-free and low-fat milk and milk products, and consume only moderate amounts of lean meats, poultry, and eggs. This approach will

help you meet your nutrient needs while maintaining energy balance. It also provides a lot of volume or bulk, which helps with satiety, increasing the sense of fullness after eating.

3) **Dramatically reduce your intake of added sugars and unhealthy fats (SoFAS). In addition, reduce sodium intake and lower your intake of refined grains, especially those that are coupled with added sugars, saturated fat, and sodium.** As I mentioned earlier, foods containing added sugars and unhealthy fats contribute excess calories to your diet and few, if any, nutrients.

The good news is that you can reach these goals with a range of dietary patterns that embrace cultural heritage, lifestyle, and food preferences, from omnivore to vegan. Try to adhere to these goals in choosing all of the foods and beverages you consume as meals and snacks throughout the day, regardless of whether they are eaten at home or away from home.

4) **Improve your health by getting enough physical activity.**

What is a healthy amount of physical activity? The committee charged with shaping the 2008 Physical Activity Guidelines for Americans looked closely at the new scientific information on physical activity and health and then helped to create science-based recommendations for the types and amounts of activity that provide the greatest benefits. Here are some of our overall findings (more details at www.fitness.gov):

- Everyone benefits from physical activity—people of all ages, from children to older adults, pregnant and postpartum women, people with disabilities, and members of every racial and ethnic group.

- A little physical activity is better than none.

- Physical activity improves health regardless of your body weight (healthy, overweight, obese).

- Both aerobic exercise and strength training improve health.

- More physical activity equals greater health benefits.

- There are many ways to be physically active: Choose to do what you like best.

As for how much is enough: Children should get 1 hour or more of physical activity every day, including a variety of moderate and vigorous activities. For adults, substantial health benefits can be gained from:

- 150 minutes per week of moderate intensity aerobic exercise, such as brisk walking OR

- 75 minutes of vigorous intensity aerobic exercise OR

- an equivalent combination of moderate- and vigorous-intensity exercise

Adults 65 years and older should adhere to the guidelines for adults or be as physically active as their fitness level and condition allows. If you are at risk for falls, you should also do exercises to maintain or improve balance.

More is better! If you want even more health benefits from physical activity, adults should increase their aerobic physical activity to 300 minutes (5 hours) a week of moderate-intensity, or 150 minutes a week of vigorous-intensity aerobic physical activity, or an equivalent combination of the two.

What is nice here is that you have a lot of flexibility in how you build physical activity into your lifestyle. You should per-form aerobic activity in bouts of at least 10 minutes. While it may be best to spread the activity throughout the week, it's fine to get all of your activity over a couple of days on the weekend. The guidelines also recommend that you do muscle-strengthening involving all of the major muscle groups on 2 or more days a week.

The report suggests that the best way to boost physical activity levels is not only through planned exercise but also through a variety of activities that expend energy throughout the day. This requires changing your home, school, work, and community environments to foster these everyday activities. What follows is a discussion of how to do that.

THE 1-DAY CHALLENGES

Creating long-lasting change is hard. As you read in Chapters 1 and 2, strong biological, cultural, and societal forces have helped to create the environment that you inhabit and shaped your behaviors within that environment. However, as most people know from experience, making short-term change is not hard. We can make a New Year's resolution and stick with it for a month or two, or we can follow a short-term diet plan, but then we usually quickly revert to our usual ways because we return to the same environment. Nothing in our surroundings has changed, so why should our long-term behavior change? This is why restructuring your personal environment is so important—when your environment changes, so does your behavior. It's not easy, but with a few successes, you'll gain confidence.

The first step toward changing your environment is to build awareness.

Three 1-Day Challenges to build awareness

Most of us have entrenched habits concerning what we eat and how much activity we get in any given day or week. Because our habits are so ingrained, most of us aren't even aware that we have them. As a first step toward making change, I've developed a series of three 1-Day Challenges aimed at building awareness of the nature of the foods you eat and the ways in which physical activity have been engineered out of your life, making you sedentary. These challenges are not long-term behavior-change strategies. They are designed as a first step to help you become aware of what you eat and how you move, so that you can become your own best expert. You will use these to build up to a 7-Day Jumpstart outlined in the next chapter.

Here are the three 1-Day Challenges:

- 1-Day No-Added-Sugars Challenge
- 1-Day No-Refined-Grains Challenge
- 1-Day 30-Minute Physical Activity Challenge

The first two challenges focus on the two food components that are by far the largest contributor to an unhealthy diet; the third is designed to help increase awareness of how to be more active throughout the day. You need not take up the challenges consecutively, but it is helpful to do them close together in time, while your mind is in the mode of discovery. Some aspects of these challenges will be easy and others, more difficult.

While I was writing this chapter, I completed each of the challenges. For me, the "No-Added-Sugars" challenge was by far the hardest. I like having a cookie after lunch and a small sweet after dinner. It wasn't easy to give these up, but it was worth it, as my level of awareness about foods that contained added sugars rose considerably. (So did my intake of fresh fruit to satisfy my sweet tooth.) When you do this challenge, you'll no doubt identify at least a few foods that you didn't realize had added sugars, such as peanut butter, many baked goods, tomato sauce, and salad dressing. Even if you find that you can't give up all the foods that contain added sugars, you'll have new understanding of how they can sneak into your diet many times a day.

1-Day No-Added-Sugars Challenge

This challenge is more difficult to execute than you might expect, because the labeling of many foods is confusing. In your typical "Nutrition Facts" label, it's hard to distinguish added sugars from sugars that are natural ingredients of the food. Luckily, there are some simple rules to help you determine if a food contains added sugar:

1. If food is a whole food (such as a piece of fruit or a vegetable) that hasn't been processed, and you haven't added any sugar yourself, then it contains no added sugars.
2. If you're eating a food with an ingredient list, look for the following terms for added sugars: sugar, sucrose, brown sugar, corn sweetener, confectioner's sugar, dextrose, fructose, fruit juice concentrate, glucose, corn syrup, high-fructose corn syrup, honey, invert sugar, lactose, maltose, maltodextrin, malt syrup, molasses, raw sugar, syrup, rice syrup, turbinado sugar, treacle, trehalose, and beet sugar.
3. If you're purchasing a food or beverage away from home and don't have access to the Nutrition Facts label or the

proprietor doesn't have an ingredients list, ask the sales personnel if any sweetener has been added. Foods likely to contain added sugars include beverages, sauces, dressings, snacks, desserts, dairy foods, and most baked goods.

Because so many foods now have excessive added sugars, there's an effort underway to change food labels to make it easier to differentiate added sugars from naturally occurring sugars—and to add to the front of a food package labeling that highlights added sugars if that food contains them. Until this change comes about, you'll need to do a little bit of deductive reasoning.

It's possible to calculate how much added sugar you get in your usual diet, though the calculation is a little tricky. If you're interested in knowing the quantity of added sugars that you consume, use the following strategy for identifying added sugars in the foods you eat:

1. If a food is not a dairy product or a product that contains fruits or vegetables, check the Nutrition Facts label. All grams of sugar that are listed are added sugars.
2. For products that contain dairy, vegetables, and fruits, you'll need to do some math to determine how many grams of sugar are added. All dairy, vegetables, and fruits naturally contain sugar. Subtract the grams of naturally occurring sugars from the grams of added sugars. Here are a few rules of thumb:
   • A cup of milk contains about 12 grams of natural sugar.
   • A cup of plain nonfat yogurt has about 19 grams of natural sugar.

- A cup of 100 percent fruit juice contains about 25 grams of natural sugar.
- A half cup cooked or whole cup raw vegetable contains about 5 grams of natural sugar.

3. Now read the Nutrition Facts label of your food product and subtract the total sugar in grams from the above. If there are more grams of sugar listed than normally occur in the food, then you can assume that sugar has been added.

4. Count the grams of added sugar in each food and total them up. To find the calorie equivalent, use the following:
   - A gram of sugar contains 4 calories.
   - A teaspoon contains 4 grams of sugar or 16 calories.

Understanding where added sugars enter your diet and how many teaspoons you typically consume each day will help you to plan how to eliminate excessive added sugars, one teaspoon at a time.

Not long ago, I decided to find out how much added sugar was in my diet. To that end, I wrote down everything I ate for a 24-hour period and then calculated the amount of added sugars. (See left-hand column in table below.) I thought the number would be low, as I'd been working to reduce them for a year or so. I was happy to see that on the recorded day, I ate only a little more than 6 teaspoons of added sugars.

The 24-hour meal plan in the right-hand column shows a different pattern. It takes my meal plan and replaces some of the foods and beverages with typical choices that contain more added sugars. While the *volume* of food per day is the same, the added sugar content, 23 teaspoons—the U.S. average for women—contains 368 additional calories. You can see what just a few changes in food choices can do to sabotage a healthy eating pattern. This illustrates the ubiquity of added sugars: They can seep into our diets from a variety of sources—many times without our even knowing it. I found this simple personal exercise highly instructive.

This chart shows all of the food I ate in one day (recorded on the left side, under the heading "low added sugars"). The column on the right reflects the same meals with just a few high-sugar substitutions (under the heading "high added sugars"). The low-added sugar meal pattern has just over six teaspoons of added sugars, while the high-added sugar one has 23 teaspoons of sugar -- the national average for women. This amounts to a large calorie difference!

Comparison of Two Different One-Day Dietary Patterns

Low Added Sugars			High Added Sugars		
Foods	Added Sugars (g)	Calories	Calories	Added Sugars (g)	Foods
Breakfast:					Breakfast:
Whole grain puffs (cup)	0	70	146	12	Honey nut cereal (cup)
2% Milk (1/2 cup)	0	65	65	0	2% Milk (1/2)
Banana (1/2)	0	45	45	0	Banana (1/2)
Orange juice (1/2 cup)	0	56	56	0	Orange juice (1/2 cup)
Black tea with 1 tsp sugar	4.2	16	120	5	Chai tea (8 oz.)
Lunch:					Lunch:
100% Whole grain bread (2 slices)	2.8	138	138	2.8	100% Whole grain bread (2 slices)
Cheddar cheese (1 oz)	0	114	114	0	Cheddar cheese (1 oz)
Tomato (1/2)	0	16	16	0	Tomato (1/2)
Peach	0	38	38	0	Peach
Ice tea with lemon (1 tsp sugar)	4.2	16	124	31	Sweetened ice tea with lemon (8 oz)
Chocolate chip cookie (1 sm)	3.4	49	49	3.4	Chocolate chip cookie (1 sm)
Snack:					Snack:
Almonds (1 oz.)	0	163	140	10	Chewy multigrain granola bar (1 oz.)
Tostitos tortilla chips (8 chips)	0	150	150	0	Tostitos tortilla chips (8 chips)
Salsa	0	36	36	0	Salsa
Dinner:					Dinner:
Salad with fresh lettuce and vegetables	0	62	62	0	Salad with fresh lettuce and vegetables
Balsamic vinegar (2 T)	0	90	282	11	French dressing (2 T)
Salmon, grilled (4.5 oz.)	0	243	243	0	Salmon, grilled (4.5 oz.)
Roasted potatoes (1 med)	0	163	163	0	Roasted potatoes (1 med)
Steamed broccoli (1/2 cup)	0	49	49	0	Steamed broccoli (1/2 cup)
Beer, lager	0	160	160	0	Beer, lager
Dessert:					Dessert:
Plain whole yogurt (3/4 cup)	0	120	150	16	Vanilla yogurt (3/4 cup)
Honey (1 teaspoon)	5.5	22			
Blueberries (1/2 cup)	0	39	39	0	Blueberries (1/2 cup)
Grams added sugars:	26			91	
Teaspoons added sugars	6.5			23	
Total calories		1,920	2,385		

1-Day No-Refined-Grains Challenge

This challenge involves identifying refined grains in your diet and eliminating them for one full day. While identifying which foods contain refined grains is fairly easy, going without them is not.

Refined grains are grains and grain products that have been processed or refined and are missing the bran, germ, and/or endosperm that contain most nutrients. Products made with refined grains include bread, pasta (including couscous), snacks, white rice, cereals, cookies, and cakes and most grained-based desserts.

Labeling regulations can make it tricky to determine whether a grain product contains whole grains. If a product says that it contains 100-percent whole grain, you can usually be assured that all of the grains are whole. Common whole grains include whole wheat, brown rice, and oats. Other less common whole grains include amaranth, barley, bulgur (cracked wheat), flaxseed, millet, quinoa, rye, spelt, wheat berries, and wild rice. However, in this country, a grain product can call itself "whole grain" if just over 50 percent of the grain it contains is whole. This means that a whole-grain bread or other grain product can contain 51 percent whole grains and 49 percent refined grains.

If a product label says "multigrain" or "whole grains" and lists several different grains, it is probably not 100-percent whole grain. Furthermore, if the product's label includes wheat flour, it likely contains little whole grain. Most whole grain or multigrain breads get their color from molasses, not from whole grains.

So, bottom line: Look for 100-percent whole grain products. Or just stick with simple oats, brown rice, and whole wheat flour for cooking and baking.

It is almost impossible to quantify the amount of refined grains in your diet, so don't worry about it. The point of this 1-Day Challenge is to become aware of where refined grains enter your daily diet and how often you consume them. If you're like most Americans, you eat only one to two servings of whole grains per day and about six to nine servings of refined grains. (A serving is 1 oz. of bread or half a cup of cereal, pasta, rice, or cooked oatmeal.)

Surprise! Clustering of the nasty stuff

After taking these two 1-Day Challenges, most people will see that added sugars and refined grains cluster together (except in the case of beverages). You may notice that unhealthy added fats also cluster with these two ingredients. Unhealthy added fats include palm oil, palm kernel oil, coconut oil, and almost all hydrogenated shortenings, many of which contain transfats. The magic troika of added sugars, refined grains, and unhealthy fats seem to make the perfect combination for tasty, convenient—and unhealthy—foods. They are the cheapest food components around and they make up the bulk of almost all grain-based desserts, snacks, and other baked goods. No wonder that grain-based desserts, including cakes, cookies, pies, doughnuts, and snack bars of all types, are the single largest contributors to calories in our diet.

1-Day Physical Activity Challenge: Build in 30 minutes of activity

This 1-Day Challenge is not as straightforward as it sounds. It's not about exercising for half an hour. Rather, the goal with this challenge involves building into your day 30 minutes of "natural" physical activity. It will also give you an idea of how much you sit during the day. If you're like most Americans, even if you exercise regularly, you tend to be very inactive the rest of the day and don't expend many calories.

What counts? There are a variety of ways to meet this challenge:

- *Stand rather than sit:* In a long meeting or at a sports event, spend part of the time standing rather than sitting.
- *Active transport:* If you commute to work, either walk or cycle part of your route. When you run an errand from home or work, walk or cycle part of the way. Whenever possible, take the stairs instead of the elevator.
- *Work time:* When possible, walk with a colleague while you talk instead of sitting in an office. Or do a "walking" errand in the middle of the work day.
- *Social time:* Instead of going to a coffee shop to visit with a friend or colleague, go for a walk. Rather than watching television with the family on Saturday morning, go for a walk or bicycle. Dance more.
- *Around the house:* rake leaves, garden, chop wood, mow the lawn with a push mower, vacuum the house.

This challenge may be easy for some and difficult for others. If possible, do it on a working day when you have less free time. The key is to identify windows in the day when you can move a little. Good luck!

ASSESSING YOUR PERSONAL ENVIRONMENT

Once you have completed the three 1-Day Challenges, you'll be more mindful of the foods you eat and when you eat them, and also how active you are throughout the day. The following assessment will help you identify the food and physical activity environment that you inhabit—in the home, at work, in your community, and in your social world. It takes only five minutes to complete. Becoming more aware of the nature of your personal environment will help you develop your plans for changing it.

Food and Physical Activity Environment Survey

Food Environment		
(Simply put a check next to all that apply.)		
Home Environment		
What do you have in your kitchen?		
	Positive	Neutral	Negative
Vegetables	___ Several fresh or frozen vegetables	___ Few (fewer than three) fresh or frozen vegetables	___ Frozen or canned vegetables combined with fat and/or salt
Fruits	___ Several fresh or frozen whole fruits	___ Few (fewer than three) fresh or frozen whole fruits	___ Frozen or canned fruits combined with added sugar/and or fat
Grains	___ 100% whole grain bread ___ 100% whole grain cereal ___ Brown rice ___ Whole oats ___ Barley ___ Quinoa ___ Bulgur ___ Wild rice ___ Wheat berries	___ Whole grain bread ___ Pasta (white) ___ White bread ___ White rice ___ Minimally sweetened cereals	___ Sugar sweetened cereals ___ Muffins ___ Biscuits ___ Doughnuts ___ Pastries
Protein foods		___ Non-lean meats	___ Fried chicken ___ Bacon ___ Sausage ___ Hot dogs ___ Bologna ___ Nuts, salted

Food Environment			
Dairy	___ Non-fat, no-sugar dairy foods such as milk and yogurt ___ Lowfat milk ___ Lowfat yogurt ___ Hard cheeses ___ Lowfat cream cheese ___ Lowfat sour cream	___ Full-fat yogurt ___ Full-fat milk	___ Ice cream ___ Yogurt with added sugars ___ Flavored milk ___ Soft cheeses ___ Prepared foods with cheese such as pizza ___ Sour cream ___ Cream cheese
Fats and oils	___ Olive oil ___ Safflower oil ___ Canola oil ___ Corn oil ___ Sesame oil ___ Soybean oil ___ Sunflower oil		___ Butter ___ Shortening with transfats ___ Coconut oil ___ Palm oil ___ Palm kernel oil
Beverages	___ Water ___ Seltzer/sparkling water ___ Unsweetened tea ___ Unsweetened coffee	___ 100% fruit juice ___ Minimally sweetened drinks with less than 50 calories/8 ounces	___ Sugar sweetened soda/pop ___ Sports drinks ___ Sweetened drinks of any kind that provide greater than 50 calories/ 8 ounces
Packaged, prepared foods	___ Packaged foods that contain no added sugar or saturated fat	___ Packaged foods that contain less that 3 grams of added sugars, low in saturated fat, and sodium	___ Snack bars ___ Meal replacements ___ Puddings ___ Sweetened gelatin foods
		___ Packaged foods that contain at least one serving of vegetables, fruits, or whole grains	
Desserts		___ Chocolate ___ Angel food cake ___ Sorbet	___ Cakes ___ Brownies/Bars ___ Cookies ___ Pies/tarts
	Count up ✓:	Count up ✓:	Count up ✓:
How do you prepare your foods?			
Cooking	___ I regularly cook meals.	___ Once or twice a week I cook meals.	___ I rarely cook meals.
Beverages	___ I rarely add cream or sugar to my tea or coffee.	___ I add one sugar and/or some milk to my tea or coffee.	___ I usually add more than one teaspoon of sugar and/or cream to my tea or coffee.
Fresh foods	___ Most of the foods I eat at home include fresh produce and minimally processed foods.	___ Some of the foods I eat at home include fresh and minimally processed foods; however I do eat some prepared and highly processed foods.	___ Most of the foods that I eat at home come from prepared meals, cans, packages and are highly processed.
	Count up ✓:	Count up ✓:	Count up ✓:

Food Environment			
How do you eat?			
At a table	___ I always eat my meals at home at a table.	___ I sometimes eat my meals at home at a table.	___ I rarely eat my meals at home at a table.
Without the television	___ I never eat with the television on.	___ I sometimes eat with the television on.	___I frequently eat with the television on.
With others, if you live with others	___Most days of the week I eat with my family or housemates.	___I sometimes eat with my family or housemates.	___I rarely eat with my family or housemates.
Regular meals	___I usually eat meals at home.	___I sometimes eat meals at home.	___I rarely eat meals at home; I usually just snack.
Consciously	___When I eat, I enjoy the foods that I am eating.	___Sometimes I'm mindful of the foods I eat.	___Several times throughout the day, I eat foods just because they are in front of me or I am bored.
	Count up ✓:	Count up ✓:	Count up ✓:
Where do you eat?	___Most days of the week I eat at least two meals at home.	___I usually have two or more meals per day away from home.	___Most of my meals are eaten away from home.
	Count up ✓:	Count up ✓:	Count up ✓:
Community Environment			
	Positive	**Neutral**	**Negative**
Where is food available in your community?	___Grocery stores with fresh produce ___Farmers' markets ___Seasonal farm stands	___Small independently owned restaurants ___Take-out establishments with healthier options	___Fast-food restaurants ___Chain restaurants ___Convenience stores ___Coffee/Pastry shops ___Superstores/box stores
Where do you shop for food?	___I regularly get my food from grocery stores and farmers' markets; and rarely from convenience stores or take-out establishments	___I buy some of my foods at a grocery store and some at a convenience store or take-out establishment	___I rarely visit a grocery store or farmers' market in my community; most of the time I buy foods at a convenience store or pick up foods at a take-out establishment
	Count up ✓:	Count up ✓:	Count up ✓:

Work Environment			
	Positive	Neutral	Negative
What is available at work?	___Refrigeration for foods brought in from home ___Food storage for healthy lunch and snacks ___Cafeteria with mostly healthy options ___When there are celebrations/events, fruits and vegetables are always available.	___Restaurants nearby with healthy options ___Sandwich and take-out shops with healthy options	___Free candy and snacks on a table or desk near your office ___There are numerous events/ celebrations at work often with only desserts and candies served. ___Vending machines with sugar-sweetened beverages ___Vending machines with candies and snacks ___Cafeteria with mostly unhealthy options ___Nearby fast-food restaurants ___Nearby chain restaurants ___Nearby coffee/ pastry shops
	Count up ✓:	Count up ✓:	Count up ✓:
How do you eat at work?	Positive	Neutral	Negative
	___I mostly bring in foods from home for lunch.	___A couple of times per week, I bring in foods from home for lunch.	___I almost always eat out for lunch.
	___I rarely eat at my desk.	___I sometimes eat at my desk.	___I always eat at my desk or in front of the computer.
	Count up ✓:	Count up ✓:	Count up ✓:
Physical Activity Environment			
Home Environment			
	Positive	Neutral	Negative
What do you have at home?	___Bicycle ___Exercise clothing ___Shoes for exercising (running, cycling, etc.) ___Home exercise equipment (treadmill, rowing machine, cycle, etc.)	___Computers in most rooms ___Leaf blowers and other convenience devices	___Television in my bedroom ___Television in my kitchen/dining area ___Non-active video games

Physical Activity Environment			
	___Portable exercise equipment (balls, weights and dumb-bells, tennis racquets, golf clubs, jump ropes, skates) ___Boating equipment ___Pedometer ___Exercise DVD ___Subscription to on-line training program ___Exercise log/calendar ___Stairs ___Dog ___Garden ___Lawn ___Axe ___Rake and other gardening tools		
	Count up ✓:	Count up ✓:	Count up ✓:
Community Environment			
	Positive	Neutral	Negative
What do you have in your community?	___Sidewalks ___Well lit streets ___Pedestrian crossings ___Bicycle lanes ___Parks ___Recreational facilities ___Community fitness centers ___Swimming pool ___Community gardens ___Rivers ___Mountains ___Close access to public transportation ___Weather is accommodating for outdoor activities		___No sidewalks ___Poorly lit streets ___No cross walks ___No public transportation ___Weather is not accommodating for outdoor activities.
	Count up ✓:		Count up ✓:

Work Environment			
	Positive	Neutral	Negative
What do you have available at work?	___There are exercise facilities at work. ___There are exercise classes offered at work. ___There are showers at work that I can use. ___There are parks or walking/running paths near work. ___ My employer pays for part of my fitness center membership.	___There are exercise facilities within a few blocks of work. ___I have access to parks or walking/running paths at work, but they are a few minutes away.	___There are no exercise facilities at work or nearby. ___There are no exercise classes offered at work. ___There are no showers at work that I can use. ___Work is not close to any parks or walking/running paths.
	Count up ✓:	Count up ✓:	Count up ✓:

There is no hard and fast way to score this assessment. In general, the more "positives" you score, the better. Having "negatives" in the food environment section is not necessarily bad. For example, I love butter and will always stock it in my house. But I also have olive oil and canola oil and use these much more often and in larger amounts. (I also always have a few small cookies on hand.) Likewise, with the physical environment, you want more positives than negatives. Ask yourself, "Do I take advantage of the physical activity resources that are available in my home, neighborhood, and at work?"

This assessment is designed to help you become more aware of your surroundings, to see where the bright spots are and where the challenges lie. You don't need to eliminate all of the negatives; rather, you want to create a healthy balance, with more positives than negatives. Your environment matters. If you find that it includes too many neutrals and negatives, the good news is that there are ways to tip the balance toward a more positive environment.

By successfully accomplishing the three 1-Day Challenges and filling out your environmental assessment, you are now "rebooted" and ready to take on a whole different way of eating and exercising. You have the tools and know-how to challenge yourself a little further, to begin to make more meaningful long-term changes in your lifestyle focused on good nutrition and physical activity. Chapters 4 and 5 will show you how to make these changes stick for a lifetime.

Chapter 4. The 7-Day Jumpstart

Now that you're more aware of exactly what you eat and your overall personal food and physical activity environment, this chapter will help you tweak it so that it's easier for you to eat and move in a healthy way over the long term. The next step is to complete a 7-Day Jumpstart, designed to guide you in this process and to help you develop your own vision of how you want to nourish yourself and be active for life.

The 7-Day Jumpstart is a single week in which you eat and move in the healthiest way possible. It builds upon the experiences you had completing the three 1-Day Challenges. Again, it isn't easy. And it isn't meant to be the model for the way you live your life from now on. Instead, it offers an opportunity to experience a pinnacle of healthy eating and activity. It's a week you can look back on for inspiration and experience to help guide you in the days, weeks, months, and years ahead. By following this jumpstart challenge, you'll reset your threshold for the taste of sugar and refined grains and begin to establish a new pattern of eating. The end goal will be to adopt a few permanent changes from those presented here, which will result in a healthier lifestyle.

7-DAY NUTRITION JUMPSTART

The first part of the 7-Day Jumpstart is focused on nutrition. This part of the jumpstart is tough, and you'll need to prepare your mind for the difficulty of following it as closely as you can. One bright note: You'll be surprised at the amount of food you can eat. Because the foods in the Jumpstart include no refined grains and no added sugar (beyond what you add from the sugar bowl), you can eat a lot of good food without taking in too many calories and still stay within the limits of healthy overall intake.

The 7-Day Jumpstart includes three general principles:

- *Focus on the foundation*: Each day you need to eat at least three whole vegetables, three whole fruits, three servings of whole grains, and three servings of protein-rich foods (greater detail provided below about amounts and choices).

- *Eat these foods in abundance*: You may eat as many whole vegetables and fruits, legumes, and whole grains as you like.

- *Avoid the two no-no's for the week:* No added sugars or refined grains.

In adhering to these three principles, you will get all of the nutrients you need—all of the vitamins, minerals, and other components to promote overall health—plus plenty of food to feel full and satisfied throughout the day. In order to follow the rules, you'll need to refer back to Chapter 3 to remind yourself how to identify added sugars and refined grains.

Why the sugar bowl?

I'm on a one-woman mission to get the sugar bowl back on the table. This may seem counterintuitive, given what you've just read about the enormous amount of added sugars in our foods these days. But the truth is, if you add your own sugar to your unsweetened foods and beverages, you'll never add as much sugar as food manufacturers add to their products. If we could get added sugars out of cereals, beverages, and prepared foods and just sweeten our food ourselves by adding our own sugar, we would be much better off. I bet you'll be surprised at how little sugar you actually need to sweeten foods to your taste. On the 7-Day Jumpstart you can add a daily total of three teaspoons of sugar to your cereal, beverage, or yogurt.

Is this a weight loss plan?

It depends. If you follow this plan for more than a week, you're likely to drop pounds, especially if you balance the calories you consume with more physical activity. In removing added sugars and refined grains from your usual food intake, you're automatically reducing the number of calories you're consuming. If you persist with this program over time, you will lose weight.

What else do I need to know to complete the jumpstart?

Try to stick with whole, minimally processed foods. It's tricky to navigate packaged foods, as it's not always easy to figure out which are free of added sugars and refined grains. Also, I would urge you to avoid consuming too many chips and other fried foods, as this can easily boost your calorie consumption to an unhealthy level (moreover, consuming them would not be in the spirit of the jumpstart).

Suggested menus for the jumpstart

The 7-Day Jumpstart is designed to make it as easy as possible to succeed. Below are three different menus for breakfast, lunch, and dinner, ranging in calories from low to moderate. Choose from this list, or if you like, make up your own menus using these as a guide. You'll see that these suggestions provide abundant food with minimal calories. When you cut refined grains and added sugars out of your diet, you can eat a lot more food, and most people find these meals very satisfying. If you choose the lower calorie menu options below, your daily total, excluding a snack, is approximately 1,200 calories; if you choose the higher calorie options, your daily total, excluding a snack, is approximately 2,000 calories. Depending upon your calorie needs, you can choose accordingly. Recipes for some of the menu items are listed after the tables.

Three Menu Options			
Breakfast (300 - 500 calories)	WHOLE GRAIN CEREAL 1 cup whole grain cereal (see list below) 1 cup 2% milk 1/2 cup sliced fruit (banana, apple, pear) or 1 cup whole berries (blueberries, strawberries, blackberries) *Approximately 300 calories* *For a higher calorie meal, choose whole milk instead of 2% milk.*	QUICK OATMEAL BREAKFAST see recipe below *Approximately 375 calories* *For a higher calorie meal, add 2 hard boiled eggs to meal.* *Approximately 525 calories*	100% WHOLE WHEAT TOAST AND EGGS 2 slices 100% whole wheat toast 1 whole egg fried in 1 tsp. butter ½ cup sliced fresh fruit *Approximately 350 calories* *For a higher calorie meal, choose 2 eggs fried in 1 tsp. butter plus ½ cup 2% milk to drink.* *Approximately 500 calories*

Three Menu Options			
Lunch (500 - 600 calories)	**CHICKEN SALAD** 2 slices whole wheat bread 1 tbs. grain mustard 3 ounces roasted chicken 3 slices of roasted red peppers 1 handful of mixed greens, shredded carrots, tomato slices (Grill sandwich if desired) *Approximately 350 calories* *For a higher calorie meal, add 1 slice full fat cheese of choice to sandwich and 1 tbs. regular mayonnaise* *Approximately 550 calories*	**SOUP AND SALAD** 1 ½ cups white bean and escarole soup prepared at home (see recipe) 1 large salad Mixed greens of your choice 2 tbs. hummus (on side) 2 tbs. goat cheese Slices of roasted red peppers 2 tbs. whole olives 1 tbs. homemade "Classic Vinaigrette" *Approximately 550 calories* *For a higher calorie meal, add ½ cup cooked beans of choice to salad* *Approximately 650 calories*	**GRILLED CHICKEN SALAD** 2 ounces grilled chicken seasoned with spices (see chart) 1 large salad 1 cup spinach or arugula 1 cup mandarin oranges ¼ cup sliced almonds 1 - 2 tbs. "Easy Classic Vinaigrette" *Approximately 450 calories* *For a higher calorie meal, add ¼ cup cheese of choice* *Approximately 600 calories*
Dinner (600 - 800 calories)	**FISH AND STEAMED VEGETABLES** 4 oz. piece of fresh fish baked with spices of choice (see chart) 1 cup steamed vegetables of choice (see chart) 1 cup brown rice 1 cup sliced fruit mixed with 1 cup full fat yogurt and 1 tsp. sugar 1 cup 2% milk *Approximately 575 calories* *For a higher calorie meal, add a 100% whole wheat dinner roll. Approximately 650 calories*	**ASIAN STIR-FRY** 6 oz. tofu cooked in wok Add some olive oil to keep from sticking with soy sauce and 1 tbs. peanut butter 1 cup cabbage (steamed) ½ broccoli (steamed) ½ cup shredded carrots ¼ cup water chestnuts 1 cup brown rice 1 cup 2% milk *Approximately 600 calories* *For a higher calorie meal, add ½ cup beans of choice and 1 additional tbs. of peanut butter to sauce.* *Approximately 800 calories*	**BEEF DINNER** 4 oz. lean beef with spices (see chart) 1 cup steamed vegetables (see chart) 1 small baked sweet potato 1 cup fruit sliced with 1 cup full fat yogurt plus 1 tsp. honey *Approximately 600 calories* *For a higher calorie meal, add a side salad with "Classic Vinaigrette" dressing plus 1 oz. cheese of choice.* *Approximately 775 calories*

The following chart offers ideas of different whole foods from which to choose within a specific food group. It includes foods with a range of calorie values. Substitute any of these for foods in the menus above. After the 7-Day Jumpstart, use these as a guide for choosing whole foods for your regular meals.

Foods: Categories & Calories

Vegetables
10 Calories
Lettuce, raw cabbage or raw spinach (1 cup) Alfalfa sprouts (1 cup) Asparagus, 4 spears, cooked Salsa (3 tbs.)
20 Calories
Celery, chopped (1 cup) Mushroom, cooked (1/2 cup) Artichokes, cooked (1/4 cup) 100% vegetable juice (1/2 cup)
30 Calories
Tomato (1 whole; 1 cup chopped) Carrot, cooked (1/2 cup) Squash, cooked (1 cup) Eggplant, cooked (1 cup) Brussels Sprouts, cooked (1/2 cup)
100 Calories
Onion, cooked (1 cup) Sweet potato, baked (1 medium)
140 Calories
Avocado (1/2 medium)
160 Calories
Potato, baked with skin (1 medium)

Fruit
60 calories
Whole fruit (apple, orange, peach) (1 medium) Banana (1 small) Grapefruit (1/2 large) Melon, diced (1 cup) Berries (blueberry, strawberry) (1 cup) Coconut, shredded (3 tbs.)
75 calories
Fruit, canned (1/2 cup) Plum (1 cup) Apricot (1 cup)
100 calories
Dried fruit (1 oz.) Mango (1 cup)
120 calories
Fruit juice (apple, orange) (1 cup) Fig (3 medium)

Grain

30 Calories

Popcorn, popped (1 cup)

50 Calories

Millet, cooked (1/4 cup)

70 Calories

100% whole wheat dinner roll (1 roll)

75 Calories

Bulgur, cooked (1/2 cup)
Wild rice, cooked (1/2 cup)

100 Calories

100% whole wheat bread (1 slice)
Brown rice, long grain, cooked (1 cup)
Barley, pearled, cooked (1/2 cup)
Whole grain cereal (3/4 cup)

150 Calories

100% whole wheat pita (1 loaf)
100% whole wheat English muffin (1 muffin)
100% whole wheat bagel (1/2 large)
Oatmeal, old-fashioned, dry (1/2 cup)
Buckwheat, cooked (1 cup)
Wheatberries, cooked (1/2 cup)

Dairy

75 calories

Goat cheese (1 oz.)

90 Calories

Milk, nonfat (1 cup)
Cottage cheese, nonfat (1/2 cup)
Ricotta cheese, low-fat (2 oz.)

100 Calories

Soy milk, unsweetened, (1 cup)
Cottage cheese, 2% fat (1/2 cup)
Ricotta cheese, whole (2 oz.)
Hard cheese, Swiss (1 oz.)

110 Calories

Hard cheese, Cheddar (1 oz.)

120 Calories

Milk, 2% fat (1 cup)
Rice milk, unsweetened, (1 cup)
Yogurt, plain low-fat (1 cup)
Cottage cheese, whole (1/2 cup)
Hard cheese, Parmesan (1 oz.)

150 Calories

Milk, whole (1 cup)
Yogurt, plain whole (1 cup)
Soft cheese, Brie, Camembert, etc. (1 oz.)

Protein
60 Calories
Peanut butter (1 tbs.)
75 Calories
Egg, large, whole Tofu, firm (1/2 cup)
100 Calories
Almond butter (1 tbs.)
120 Calories
Beans, Pinto (1/2 cup) Beans, Black (1/2 cup) Lentils (1/2 cup) Edamame beans (1/2 cup)
140 Calories
Fish, light colored (flounder, cod) (4 oz.) Seafood (shrimp, scallop, clam) (4 oz.) Poultry, light meat without skin (4 oz.)
160 Calories
Nuts (1 oz.)
220 Calories
Fish, dark colored (salmon, bluefish) (4 oz.) Poultry, dark meat without skin (4 oz.) Beef, lean (round, loin, flank) (4 oz.) Pork, lean (tenderloin, round) (4 oz.) Lamb, lean (4 oz.)
300 Calories
Beef (chuck, hamburger) (4 oz.) Pork (chops, spare ribs) (4 oz.) Lamb (chop) (4 oz.)
Fats
60 calories
Half and Half (3 tbs.)
100 calories
Butter (1 tbs.) Mayonnaise (1 tbs.) Heavy Cream (2 tbs.)
120 calories
Olive oil (1 tbs.) Canola oil (1 tbs.)
140 calories
Oil and Vinegar salad dressing (2 tbs.)

Sweets
16 Calories
Maple syrup (1 tsp.) Brown sugar (1 tsp.) Sugar (1 tsp.)
20 Calories
Honey (1 tsp.)
Alcohol
60 Calories
Liquor (Gin, Rum, Whiskey, Vodka) (1 fl oz.)
90 Calories
Wine, red (3.5 fl oz.) Wine, white (3.5 fl oz.)
100 Calories
Beer, light (12 oz.) Liqueur (1 fl oz.)
150 Calories
Beer, regular (12 oz.)

A few recipes

Here are a few recipes mentioned in the menus above.

Quick Oatmeal

Ingredients:

- 1/2 cup old-fashioned oatmeal

- 1/2 cup 2 percent milk

- 1 tbsp. walnuts (or other nuts)

- 1 tbsp. sunflower seeds

- 1/2 cup fresh mixed berries or fresh frozen berries

Preparation: Heat oatmeal and milk in microwave or on stove-top until heated through or pour milk over oatmeal and refrigerate overnight. Add nuts, seeds and berries just before eating.

Escarole and White Bean Soup
Ingredients:

- 1/4 cup extra-virgin olive oil

- 1 large onion, chopped

- 1 cup halved cherry tomatoes

- 1/2 cup finely chopped celery

- 1/2 cup finely chopped carrot

- 1/4 cup chopped garlic

- 2 tsp. Italian seasoning, or 1 tbsp. each chopped fresh basil and oregano

- 1/2 tsp. freshly ground pepper

- 2 14-oz. cans vegetable broth or chicken broth

- 2 15-oz. cans cannellini beans, rinsed

- 1 head escarole, chopped

- 1/2 cup freshly shredded hard Italian cheese, such as Parmesan, Romano or Asiago

Preparation: Heat oil in a dutch oven over medium heat. Add onion, tomatoes, celery, carrot, garlic, Italian seasoning and pepper and cook, stirring often, until the vegetables begin to soften and the onion is translucent, about 10 minutes. Add broth, bring to a simmer and cook, stirring often, until vegetables are tender. Stir in beans and escarole and cook, stirring often, until the escarole is just tender, about 5 minutes. Serve with a sprinkle of cheese.

Classic Vinaigrette
Ingredients:

- 1/2 cup extra virgin olive oil
- 2 tbsp. – 1/4 cup balsamic vinegar or white wine vinegar (based on your preference)
- 1 tbsp. whole grain mustard
- Cracked black pepper to taste
- Salt to taste
- 1 tsp. honey
- 1/2 tsp. dried tarragon or basil (optional)

Preparation: Blend all ingredients except olive oil, then slowly pour in olive oil and whisk together while pouring.

Spice Chart
Spices are a great way to provide flavor for foods without adding significant calories. Below are suggestions for spices that go well with some of the basic foods in the menus.

Seasonings for robust flavor		
Beans	**Tofu**	**Fish**
• dill	• soy sauce	• lemon
• cilantro	• curry	• basil
• rosemary	• pineapple	• curry powder
• sage	• onion	• dill
• onion	• lemon	• garlic
• garlic	• pepper	• nutmeg
	• tomato	• paprika
	• paprika	• parsley
	• cayenne	• sage
		• rosemary
Chicken and turkey	**Lean meats (includ-ing beef, pork, lamb)**	**Lean ground meats**
• curry powder	• allspice	• allspice
• ginger	• basil	• basil
• lemon	• caraway seed	• dry mustard
• dry mustard	• bay leaves	• nutmeg
• nutmeg	• curry powder	
• rosemary	• garlic	
• sage	• lemon juice	
	• mustard	
	• onion	
	• paprika	
	• parsley	
	• rosemary	
	• sage	
	• thyme	
	• turmeric	

Whole Grain Cereals

Cereals are an easy, convenient way to start the day, but most contain a lot of added sugars. Below is a list of commercial or packaged cereals that have either no added sugar or very little (less than 3 grams):

• Post Shredded Wheat

• General Mills Cheerios (1 gram added sugars)

• Bob's Red Mill 10 Grain Hot Cereal

- Bob's Red Mill Grains & Nuts Hot Cereal

- Kashi 7 Whole Grain Cereals Nuggets (3 grams of added sugars)

- Kashi 7 Whole Grain Cereals Puffs

Dried Beans and Whole Grains

Some people are put off by the trouble of preparing whole grains and legumes. The truth is, they're easy to prepare; they just take a little longer to cook. All this means is that you have to think ahead. The first thing I do when I get home is to start cooking brown rice. Then I change, relax, and prepare the rest of the dinner. By the time I'm done with the other dinner preparations, the rice is ready.

For easy whole grain and bean preparation, follow the instructions below.

Dried Beans

- Soak all dried beans except lentils, split peas and black-eyed peas.
  Overnight soak – cover beans with water and soak overnight, 6-8 hours.
  Quick soak – bring water to a boil, add beans and return to a boil; remove from heat and let soak for 2-3 hours.

- Drain beans and rinse in a strainer before cooking.

- To cook, cover beans with fresh water and bring to a boil, then simmer for approximately 45 minutes. (Cooking times vary based on type of beans.)

- Beans keep well in the refrigerator for up to 5 days. You can also freeze cooked beans for later use.

Whole Grains

- Whole grains are prepared much like rice. Cooking times vary; follow instructions in cookbook or on package.
- Soaking whole grains may help to speed up the cooking time. Some grains must be soaked overnight before cooking, including rye, spelt berries and wheatberries.
- Whole grains keep well in the refrigerator for up to 5 days. Use them in soups, salads or as a side dish.

While we're on the subject of whole grains, here is one more recipe—among my favorites. It comes from my book, *Strong Women Eat Well*, written with Judy Knipe. This recipe is easy to make, and my children and husband love it.

Wheatberries with Fruit and Honey-Orange Salad
Wheatberries are a whole grain that can be purchased at most natural foods stores. I like this grain salad best made with soft wheatberries, which cook up to a beautiful pale color and a tender but crunchy texture. The dish is delicious served by itself or as an accompaniment to meats, fish and poultry. I also love it for breakfast, topped with some yogurt. The recipe makes 3 1/2 - 4 cups, about eight servings.
Ingredients:

- 1 cup summer (soft) wheatberries
- 1 orange for zest and juice
- 1/2 cup dried cranberries, coarsely chopped

- 1/2 cup dried (unsulfured) apricots, cut into thin slivers
- 6 tbsp. pine nuts
- 4 tsp. honey
- Salt to taste

There are two ways to soak wheatberries. Soak them overnight in water, covering the wheatberries by an inch. Alternatively, you can place them in a heavy medium-size saucepan, add water to cover by at least an inch, and bring to a boil. Cover the pan, turn off the heat, and let the berries sit for two hours.

Once the wheatberries are soaked by either method, drain them, return to the pan, and cover with at least an inch of fresh water. Bring to a boil, lower the heat, and simmer the berries covered for about 30 minutes, or until the grain is cooked but still crunchy. Add salt to taste 10 minutes before the grain is done. Drain the wheatberries and transfer to a bowl. You will have a generous 2 1/2 cups.

Using a vegetable peeler, remove the zest from the orange in long strips. Cut 8 or 9 strips of it into very thin slivers, then cut the slivers into tiny dice. Add to the wheatberries with the cranberries, apricots, and pine nuts. Squeeze the 4 tbsp. of juice from the orange into a small bowl, whisk in the honey, and add to the salad. Mix well and taste for salt. (Salt added in very small amounts brings out the flavor of the fruit.)

Serve warm, at room temperature, or cold.

7-DAY JUMPSTART - PHYSICAL ACTIVITY CHALLENGE

The second part of the 7-Day Jumpstart is straightforward. The goal is to meet the 2008 Physical Activity Guidelines for one week. This can be achieved through a variety of approaches: You can meet the challenge through planned, intentional exercise, by actively transporting yourself for work or errands, or through play, dance, or sports. The choice is up to you.

Physical activity 7-day goal
150 minutes of moderate OR 75 minutes of vigorous aerobic activity

Here are a few examples of how to meet the challenge:

Planned exercise: Three days per week, twenty-five minutes per session of vigorous activity, such as running, biking, or swimming.

Active transport: Thirty minutes per day, five days per week of commuting to and from work by walking or biking.

Play, dance, sports, or work: One hour a week of dancing and one hour of playing doubles tennis, as well as 30 minutes per week of raking leaves.

Weekend warrior: A two-and-a-half hour hike on a Saturday or Sunday.

What about strength training?
Ideally, the physical activity part of your 7-Day Jumpstart includes strength training two to three days per week. This can be accomplished by going to a fitness center and lifting weights, working out at home with simple dumbbells and ankle weights, using your own body weight for push-ups, sit-ups, wall squats, and lunges, or by doing other recreational activities such as rock climbing. Activities around the house and yard such as chopping wood or doing heavy yard work

can also count as strengthening activities. My website and several of my previous books contain simple strength training programs that you can easily follow at home (see www.strong-women.com).

CREATE YOUR OWN PHILOSOPHY FOR HEALTHY LIVING

You've completed the 7-Day Jumpstart. You've learned a lot about your own habits and what needs changing. Now is the time to develop your own principles for healthy living, for how you wish to nourish yourself and stay active in the long run.

A Nutrition-for-Life Philosophy

In building a healthy diet, I suggest that you let the planet be your guide. Be mindful of your choices and don't take good nutrition for granted. Choose a foundation of real foods, grown from the earth. Take the time to truly enjoy the foods you eat. A nutrition philosophy should reflect who you are as an individual. Make sure that you embrace your individuality. Find inspiration from your cultural heritage, family traditions, and life experiences to guide your food choices.

Here is my nutrition philosophy for life:

1. The planet is my guide

Eat foods from the earth. The most healthful and nutritious foods come directly from the earth. Our current food supply does not encourage this way of eating, so it takes some effort. When choosing foods, I ask myself "Where did this come from?" I want to be sure I know the answer. I focus on foods that are whole, minimally processed, and with little packaging.

If there's an ingredient list, I choose foods that contain few ingredients and make sure that I recognize all of them.

Shift toward more plant-based foods. Over the past few years I've worked to move toward a diet that is primarily plant-based. Plant foods such as vegetables, fruits, beans, nuts, and seeds are nutrition powerhouses and are naturally healthful. I'm fortunate in that my brother and sister-in-law manage a small organic farm in New Hampshire. In addition to fruits and vegetables, they also have sheep, pig, and chickens. Each year my family and I purchase half a pig, a lamb, and about twenty chickens and eat this meat all year, which works out to about one meal of meat per week. The meat is delicious, and because I know and trust the source, I'm assured that the animals have been treated well. Few people have this kind of direct access to an organic farm, but more local farmers are selling meat that they've raised in a responsible fashion. I encourage you to seek out these local farmers and support them.

I also eat fresh fish about once a week, as well as eggs and dairy. I try to limit my dairy to good-quality yogurt, cheese, and milk. I do my best to choose foods that are in season and haven't traveled far to arrive on my plate.

2. Nourish my body for peak health

Fuel for life. I strive to keep my body nourished with quality fuels. Because the brain and body need continual nourishment to work at peak performance, I eat periodically throughout the day—breakfast, lunch, afternoon snack, and dinner. Nourishing myself often gives me the energy to accomplish the tasks of daily life and to engage in the vigorous physical activity I enjoy.

Maintain energy balance. I know that a healthy lifestyle is about balance. In nutrition, balance is maintained by making judicious choices in both the quality and the quantity of the foods I eat. I try to consume mostly high-quality, nutritious foods and have learned to balance how much I eat with my level of physical activity. As I get older, this has gotten more difficult, but maintaining a healthy weight means a lot to me, so I consider it worth the effort.

3. Be mindful and thankful

Make time for meals. I try to set aside time in my day to eat well. Taking even just a few extra minutes allows me to be present—and thankful—for my meals.

Savor the experience. Meals are not only about what you eat, but also *how* you eat. I try to fully engage in the experience of my meals: the food, the conversation, and the environment. Some key rules help me abide by this. I always enjoy dinner at a table with my family, with the television and computer off. I'm working harder to do the same during my lunches at the office, but it doesn't always happen.

Consider the impact. I'm very aware that the impact of my food choices goes beyond my personal health; it extends to my family and to the environment as a whole. I try to choose wisely. I look for foods that are sustainably grown, produced, and packaged. I believe that we can nourish our bodies and be gentle on the environment at the same time. I understand that this costs a little more, so I choose carefully where I spend extra money. However, I still spend less on food than do most people living in developed countries because food in the U.S. is cheaper.

Create your own nutrition philosophy

Now you know my nutrition philosophy. What's yours? I encourage you to take time to envision your ideal food lifestyle.

Think about the following questions:

- What types of foods would you like to eat?

- Where would you like to purchase your food?

- How would you like to prepare your meals?

- With whom would you like to enjoy your meals?

Write down your vision of an ideal food lifestyle. Make it as detailed as you like. Keep it somewhere, in a private or public space where you can see it on a regular basis and will be sure to notice it nearly every day. It will serve as a reminder of where you're going on your personal journey.

Ideal Food Lifestyle

My Ideal Food Lifestyle
I would like to eat more of these foods:
I would like to eat fewer of these foods:
I would like to purchase my food from the following places:
I would like to prepare my meals/snacks in the following ways:
I would like to be enjoying my meals (where and with whom): Breakfast: Lunch: Dinner: Other:

A Physical-Activity-for-Life Philosophy

Having completed the 7-Day Jumpstart, you know what it takes to meet the 2008 Physical Activity Guidelines for Americans. I encourage you to determine the best way for you to continue doing so, to help you stay healthy for life. The beauty of physical activity is that you can be really creative in how you meet the guidelines. You don't even have to put your sneakers on if you don't want to, as you can wear comfortable shoes while you meet the guidelines by transporting yourself from one place to another. You have the power and knowledge to create a lifestyle that has plenty of physical activity. You just need to be deliberate and intentional. I suggest that you target activities you enjoy the most—that way you will be more likely to stick with them over time.

Here is my physical-activity philosophy for life:

1. Seek out active transport as often as possible.

If I can walk or bike somewhere instead of drive, I will do so. I'm lucky that I live just a couple of blocks from the train station. Most days of the week, I take the train to work. While the station near my home is only two blocks away, the station where I get off for work is a 23-minute walk right through downtown Boston to my office. On days that I walk to and from the train station, I get about 45-50 minutes of walking built right into my day. So even on days when I don't have time to fit in a formal exercise session, I can still be very active. While this isn't vigorous activity, it is moderate and very pleasurable. And the walking helps me to relieve stress and reflect on my day. Wherever I am, I seek out these opportunities for walking or biking. Many days this is the only type of activity I get.

2. Break a sweat at least three times a week.

I enjoy vigorous exercise. I love to run, cycle, hike, cross-country ski, and swim. For optimal health, I try to break a sweat three times per week. (I use "break a sweat" as a rule of thumb, as it is a good indication of the intensity of a workout.) Research is clear that vigorous physical activity offers great benefits.

3. Play, dance, sports, work, and seeking out active fun.

I like to seek out other opportunities to be active during the week: going to the rock-climbing gym, chopping wood, shoveling snow, and taking walks with friends. While I would love to dance more, I only do this once or twice a year. This year I plan to dance at every chance I get. Several times a season, I help my husband with the yard work. Friends of mine have great fun playing soccer or tennis in adult leagues.

Create your own physical activity philosophy

Take the time to envision your ideal physical activity lifestyle. Think about the following questions:

- What activities do you enjoy most?

- Where in your typical day can you add in more light and moderate activity?

- Is there a way for you to increase your activity by active transport, such as commuting or doing errands?

- Is it possible for you to get some vigorous activity at some point during the week?

- Are there physical chores around the house that you actually enjoy and could do more often?

- Can you have more fun by dancing more or playing active sports with friends?

Write down your vision of your ideal physical activity lifestyle. Use the chart below to outline your vision. Make it as detailed as you like.

Ideal Active Lifestyle

My Ideal Active Lifestyle
Each week I would like to accumulate: _____minutes of moderate activity _____minutes of vigorous activity
I will accomplish this goal by (type and frequency): Planned exercise: Active transport: Playing, dancing, sports, work, and having active fun:
I am feeling adventurous and would like to take on a new goal for physical activity:
During the different seasons I plan to participate in different sports and fun activities:
I would like to limit my television and other sedentary time to:

CHANGE YOUR SURROUNDINGS: SUPPORT YOUR NEW VALUES AND GOOD HABITS

Now that you've completed the 7-Day Jumpstart, you understand what it takes to eat well and move more. You've experienced what it's like to eat a diet based on whole, real foods and minimally on prepared or convenience foods. You've experienced what it feels like to meet the 2008 Physical Activity Guidelines for Americans. (You're among the 5 percent of Americans who actually follow the guidelines.) You've shaped your own personal philosophy of nutrition and physical activity.

This part of the book offers suggestions for reshaping your food and physical activity environment to support your values and make it easier to sustain some of the good habits you experienced during the 7-Day Jumpstart, so they become a regular part of your life. Pick and choose what works for you. Be creative.

A note about values and priorities: People often say they don't have time to prepare their own food or to exercise properly. But consider this: Many people spend up to four hours a day watching TV or on Facebook. Why isn't it possible to carve out 30 minutes for cooking or physical activity? Likewise, people often complain that good, whole food is too expensive and yet they don't think twice about spending $200 per month on phone, internet, or cable service. I think we all need to look closely at where we choose to spend our time and money and make good eating and exercise a top priority.

Bring in the good stuff

The first step in creating a healthy home food environment is to bring in good food and minimize unhealthy food. In short, shop differently. It's likely that you're the gatekeeper, not only for yourself but also for your family. Whatever you bring into the house is what you and your family will eat. What you want is a refrigerator, pantry, and freezer stocked with healthy food. Slowly work toward having more whole foods, including vegetables, fruits, whole grains, raw or dry-roasted nuts and seeds, fish, quality dairy, and lean meats. And work toward stocking no sugar-sweetened beverages, fewer snack foods and cereals with added sugars and refined grains, and fewer desserts. It's simple: If a food or beverage is in your house, it will likely get eaten; if it isn't, it won't.

In many communities, the food environment is rapidly changing. People are putting a lot of work into increasing access to healthier foods, with more farmers' markets and greater emphasis on local foods. The problem is that most communities still have abundant sources of unhealthy foods, especially foods laden with added sugars, refined grains, and unhealthy fats. These are found in corner convenience stores, gas stations, coffee shops, pharmacies, and just about any-where people shop.

We live one block from a major crossroad in our neighbor-hood. The four corners have one convenience store, two coffee shops, and a gas station. All four stores sell foods containing literally a ton of added sugars and refined grains. A while ago, I walked through all of them and found that the total amount of space devoted to whole food (besides coffee beans) was one small basket of fifteen bananas at the convenience store and some yogurt with fruit at one of the coffee shops. There were no 100-percent whole grains, no vegetables, no legumes. Out of four establishments, only fifteen bananas and few cups of yogurt. Wow! Luckily, we have a fish store and a small grocery store only a block farther down the street, and our super-market is just another block beyond that. Even for my family members, who are motivated to eat well, that corner with the four shops wins out much of the time.

In reshaping your food environment, identify which shops carry the healthiest food and try to buy there. If possible, move away from box stores or larger superstores—or at least be vigi-lant about the foods that you purchase there. Because these stores sell packaged foods in bulk, people end up purchasing multiple boxes or bags of unhealthy foods and little fresh produce (although some superstores are beginning to offer more fresh produce and organic foods).

At the grocery store, limit your shopping to the outer aisles, where the produce and dairy items are displayed and stay away from the middle aisles, which tend to hold highly processed foods. Go for what's ripe and fresh and try for variety.

When possible, buy fresh foods that are local. Try to locate local sources of fresh produce by talking with your friends and reading the local newspaper. Find out if there are any farmers' markets or farm stands nearby. Does your nearest food market carry plenty of fresh produce? Do you have a local source for farm-raised meats? Can you get a share at a local CSA (community supported agriculture)? More communities are increasing access to local fresh produce. Buying from these sources not only supports your health, but supports the local economy and environment as well.

Buying local fresh produce means being flexible about the seasons. During the summer and fall, access to local farmers' markets may be easier than in the winter and early spring. Take advantage of the seasons. Our family eats more fresh foods in the summer and fall and more frozen foods in the winter—but in the winter months, we try to find the best fresh foods even if they aren't local, such as citrus, carrots, and broccoli.

Before you step foot in the store or market, make a grocery list. It will go a long way toward ensuring that you bring in the good stuff and will help to reduce impulse buying.

Healthy foods insight

Where you place food in the house greatly influences what you eat. If there's a plate of cookies on the kitchen table, you and your family will go for these; if it's a bowl of sliced fruit or vegetables, that's what you'll eat. You can cut up healthy food that needs to be refrigerated and place it in a container in the front of the refrigerator for easy access.

Bottom line: Put healthy foods in sight; make less healthy foods less visible and less accessible. This really works.

Size matters

When you snack or eat a meal, prepare smaller portions. And whatever you do, don't put out large family-style platters at meals. When large amounts of food are regularly placed on the table for easy access, people eat more. Get in the habit of serving smaller portions. If you or your family members need to go back for seconds, that's fine. One interesting experiment showed that adults eat less when given smaller servings and told they can go back for more, than they do if they are given heaping helpings the first time around.

Eating from smaller plates and bowls and drinking from smaller glasses also helps you eat less. Unfortunately, our plates, bowls, and glasses have increased in size over the past few decades. If possible, go for small.

Where we eat matters

If I could change one thing about Americans' eating habits, it would be getting people to eat at tables. We eat food in the strangest places: in the car, in front of the television, at our desks, walking down the street, standing up at the counter. Only occasionally do we eat at a table. All of this contributes to mindless eating. When we don't savor and enjoy our food in an appropriate setting, we tend to eat more. Think about where you eat, and whenever possible, eat at a table.

Grass to gardens

Home gardens have gained popularity over the past couple of years. Consider growing some of your own food, even if you have only a small yard or porch. Your local cooperative extension or land-grant university can provide you with guidance. Tomatoes, carrots, lettuce, and basil are just a few of the foods and herbs that can be grown quite easily in a window box or pot on the porch. This will get you in a mindset of procuring and enjoying fresh food and increase your mindfulness and appreciation of it.

Neelam Sharma's effort to convert lawns to vegetable and fruit gardens in South Central L.A. is a very inspiring story with great results. If people can grow their own food in South Central L.A., they can do it almost anywhere (see Chapter 7).

Cook!

There is no doubt about it: When we eat foods that we have cooked ourselves, we eat more healthfully. In the past few decades, however, with more women working and juggling multiple responsibilities, we have been cooking less. In fact, as noted in Chapter 2, we now spend much less of our disposable income on foods eaten at home. The market has responded to these demographic shifts by providing more and more cheap and convenient foods.

Not long ago, our family moved. The month before, we were overwhelmed with packing and organizing our stuff. We ate out a lot or bought more take-out. At first I was delighted at not having to cook, but after a few days, I tired of the food. While we did our best to choose our take-out and restaurant meals wisely, we still couldn't get the quantity of vegetables and whole grains we enjoy. After we arrived at the new house, the first thing we did was to dig into the kitchen boxes so we could get back to cooking. My husband and I made a pact to eat out less. To that end, we have found some simple main dishes that we can whip up for supper faster than ordering take-out.

Think about the meals you enjoy cooking. Consider taking a cooking class with friends to learn new recipes that are easy and delicious. The key is to have a few staples on hand that you can use to make a quick meal in a pinch.

Be mindful of the foods you eat at work

If creating change at home is difficult, creating change outside your home is even harder. Most of us spend the majority of our days at work, where we have even less control over our food environment than we do at home.

The best way to improve what you eat at work is to bring in your own food. Foods you prepare are almost always going to be healthier than what you can buy at work. When you're making dinner the night before, make a little extra and bring in the leftovers.

If you can't bring your own food, identify the healthiest lunch venues. Look for a place that will make your favorite sandwich on 100-percent whole grain bread, or will prepare salads without a lot of extra dressing, or offer entrées in small portions with a generous helping of vegetables.

Casual food in the workplace can also be a problem: the M&Ms at the administrative assistant's desk, the pretzels next to the microwave, the cake that shows up every week for a baby shower or retirement celebration. The calories from these "casual foods" add up. Try to avoid these temptations.

Finally, work days are long. It's unreasonable to think that you can go from lunch to dinner without a snack. Don't count on the vending machine; instead, consider bringing in a yogurt or a small whole-grain sandwich as an afternoon snack. I try to tuck into my purse a good-size banana and some almonds for my snack. These satisfy my sweet tooth and sustain me until dinnertime.

Eating away from home

Restaurants and other eating venues are part of our personal food environment. This is true now more than ever. Every day, most of us consume at least one or two meals away from home. Choose wisely. Pick local restaurants or take-out places near your home that have the healthiest food, with whole grains and large portions of vegetables, for instance. Be creative. And be assertive with the restaurant staff. What is put before you is most likely what you will eat, so ask the waiter to skip the basket of white bread. When you order, ask for half of the meat portion and twice the vegetables, or split a main course with your dining partner.

Creating an active home environment

Managing the television and other electronic devices will go a long way toward creating a more active household. There are many other ways to make your home more conducive to physical activity. If you like exercising at home, create a space for exercise and buy an exercise mat and some weights. (In our basement, I have an exercise ball that I use while watching a few innings of the Red Sox in the evening.) Install a pull-up bar in a commonly used doorway. If you like using stationary exercise equipment, look around for a good-quality, second-hand piece of equipment. Get a couple of exercise videos that you enjoy and can easily pop in the DVD player. Subscribe to an online exercise prescription that makes it easy to follow a program. One of my colleagues subscribes to an online yoga site with short and long programs that she can tap into anytime, anywhere.

To create an active home environment, think about the activities that you like the most and nudge yourself to do them. Think about your most common sedentary activities at home (besides sleeping) and consider how to minimize them.

Locating physical activity opportunities outside the home

After completing the personal environment questionnaire, you should have a good idea of opportunities available in your community and near your workplace for recreation and physical activity, both indoor and outdoor. Look at programs offered by your employer. Seek out local fitness centers and smaller fitness programs, as well as community centers. Consider places outdoors where you can easily walk or run, such as local parks, conservation land, and local high schools, which may have tracks, walking trails, safe streets for cycling, and sidewalks.

Choosing active transport

Children and adults alike tend to get the most activity in their days by transporting themselves from one place to another. Lately, much of that transport is by way of car. *Active transport* is moving yourself on your own steam—by walking or cycling, for instance. Even when you take a car, there's often opportunity for some kind of active transport. Consider walking or biking part of your route. If you park in a garage near your office, avoid taking the shuttle van and walk instead. At least once or twice a week, do an errand by foot or bicycle. If you take public transportation, get off the bus or train a few stops before your destination and walk the rest of the way. All of this adds up quickly.

Managing the television

One of the biggest obstacles to eating well and creating an active home is the way we use the television. Many American households watch television while eating their meals, which contributes to the nation's expanding waistline. When we eat with the television on, we don't monitor our intake. Turning off the television when you eat will help you to be more mindful of the food you're eating and to consume a little less.

Think about where you place your televisions. Be aware that having one in the bedroom of children is *strongly* associated with childhood obesity. For adults, it contributes to poor sleep, which may be a contributing factor in overweight and obesity.

In our house, our television is currently in our basement, so we have to go downstairs to watch it. When the children were young, it was in the living room, and I found that they watched too much because it was always there right in front of them. When we moved it, television viewing in our whole family declined precipitously. Out of sight, out of mind. This may be too draconian for many people, but do consider where the television is in the house and how much you watch it. Watching less will help you eat less and be more physically active. The same goes for computers and other electronic devices that offer television and other programming. Turn off all devices when you eat. It's just good practice.

For many people, extra calories sneak into their diets during after-dinner TV-viewing, when they experience an almost Pavlovian reflex to reach for the brownies, cookies or cake. The secret is keeping your body busy: folding laundry, knitting or doing needlepoint, doing yoga, lifting weights or doing squats.

Reducing the amount of time you spend in front of the television or the glowing monitor frees up time for a more active lifestyle. By simply switching off your television, DVD player, stereo and computer more, you will spontaneously become more active and improve your energy balance.

ENVISION THE CHANGE YOU HOPE TO ACCOMPLISH

When thinking about how you wish to change your environment, envision what your life will look like after the shift. Picture yourself accomplishing your goal. Imagine a personal environment in which it's easier for you to live a healthy lifestyle. Who will be there to support you? Who may attempt to sabotage your efforts along the way? How will you handle this? What will your pantry and refrigerator look like? Where will you be walking? Think through as many details as you can. Write them down. As you go along, keep track of your successes and challenges. Your experience will help guide your continuing efforts to change.

Focus on only one or two changes at a time

The options for creating change in your personal environment are nearly limitless. That's the good news. But research shows us that when people work on too many changes at once, they usually fail. It's the rare person, indeed, who can quit smoking, cut down on drinking, lose weight, start flossing her teeth, and run a marathon all at once. The vast majority of us have greater success at long-term change if we focus on one or two goals. For this reason, I strongly recommend that you choose only one food-related change and one physical-activity-related change, and commit yourself to making these changes for only one month.

Listed below are specific areas of your personal food and physical activity environment where you might decide to tackle change:

Ideas for change in your food environment:

- Change where you shop (buy more foods from a farmers' market and less from a superstore or box store) so that you bring home more fresh produce and fewer processed foods.

- Make healthier foods more accessible (put more fruit on the kitchen counter).

- Reduce portion size (make smaller serving sizes and use smaller plates, bowls, and glasses).

- Examine your routines for unhealthy habits. For instance, do you walk or drive past the bakery or coffee shop and have trouble resisting the lure of a donut or a grande café latte? Try changing your route to avoid temptations.

- Plant a small garden in your yard or on your porch.

- Cook more.

- Take more home-cooked food to work.

- Eat only at a table and never in the car or at your desk.

- Eat out less often.

Ideas for change in your physical activity environment:

- Watch less television. Move the TV out of the family room, kitchen, or bedroom. Have a "television off" rule while eating.

- Subscribe to an online exercise program that offers you flexibility.

- Place an exercise mat near your television or in a space that you occupy a lot.

- Take advantage of your natural resources, parks, and recreation areas in your neighborhood.

- Increase your active transport to work and for errands.

- Join a community exercise program.

- Walk with a friend.

- Do more yard work and outdoor chores.

- Dance more.

Only you know what will work best for you. Take a look at the suggestions in this chapter or create your own list. Consider each change. Which will have the greatest impact? Which do you have the most confidence that you'll succeed in? Choose two specific changes—one related to food and one, to physical activity. Decide how many times per week you want to do them. It's important to commit fully to the two goals and to have confidence in your ability to succeed in making the change for a specific amount of time. With each success, you'll have more confidence, which will make it easier to make subsequent changes.

After a month, take a critical look at your efforts. This is essential. Only by considering what worked—and why—will you be able to make other changes necessary to create a truly healthy personal food and physical activity environment. Until our world changes—until our larger food and physical activity environment is such that healthy choices are relatively effortless—each of us must alter our own personal environments to support healthy living. This isn't easy, but it's a great way to make lasting positive change in your own life and to powerfully influence others.

Making permanent change is difficult. Fortunately, research shows that it's far easier when we surround ourselves with supportive friends, family, coworkers, etc. The key is harnessing our social networks to help us maintain healthy change. The next chapter offers suggestions on how to do just that.

Chapter 5. Friends for Life

Martha and Deanne accomplished their remarkable changes by creating new environments for themselves. Martha's change was precipitated by her move from Atlanta to Denver. For Deanne, the changes came once she finally "flipped her switch" and decided to reshape her surroundings. However, in both instances, the key to success lay in adopting new networks of friends and colleagues.

It's nearly impossible to make change alone. The key to living well is surrounding yourself with a social network that supports the lifestyle you want to lead. Martha found buddies to walk with and a neighbor to join her for regular spinning classes. Deanne developed new friendships through running groups and races. Neither Martha nor Deanne could have succeeded in their efforts without these "friends for life."

We're just beginning to understand how profoundly we're affected by our social networks. The emerging research in this area is intriguing. In Chapter 1, you read about how social networks strongly influence body weight and health-related lifestyle behaviors, and that there seems to be a contagion effect of high body weight among close friends. We can't help but imitate others; this is true for adults as well as children. As a scientist involved in obesity prevention research, I'm fascinated by this phenomenon. I know from my own experience that the company I keep has a major influence on my actions.

Some exciting new research supports this idea. One ten-month study conducted by colleagues at Brown University tested the hypothesis that participating in a weight loss program with a strong network of friends would help an individual maintain long-term weight loss. The investigators designed the study to look at whether creating a "new friends" network, working together with existing friends, or doing the program on one's own would best support long-term positive change. The findings clearly demonstrated that people who underwent behavior change to improve body weight and nutrition did much better when they had friends completing the program with them. It didn't matter whether the friends were new or old.

Of course, it's important to understand that the impact of our social networks can be a serious double-edged sword: They can either support or hinder healthy lifestyle habits. As we've seen, they can even foster the spread of overweight and obesity.

I believe that we can turn around the epidemic of overweight in this country with the help of the very same social networks that fuel it. The question is: How do we harness their power for a positive outcome?

HOW DO SOCIAL NETWORKS AFFECT YOUR HEALTH?

A social network consists of a group of people and the connections between them. The network can be just two people, a few people, or a lot of people. It can include friends, family, colleagues, or people from a group such as a congregation. Most individuals have about six people with whom they are closely connected in a network.

Research suggests that social networks may support or thwart healthy behaviors in three key ways:

1. *Social networks provide practical and emotional support*.

Social networks are a great way of locating resources that support healthy behavior. A good example is a parent network, where parents share information about a restaurant that offers healthy meals for kids or wisdom on the best pediatrician in town or news about a new yoga studio opening up down the street or an easy way to prepare whole grains. Networks may also provide direct practical support for achieving a healthy behavior. Someone you know knows someone who can provide childcare, so that you can get to the gym a few times a week; a friend offers you a ride to spinning classes; a neighbor steps in to cook a meal for your family, giving you time to walk.

Friends, family, and colleagues can also offer empathy and understanding when it comes to the challenges of making healthy change. They can act as a nonjudgmental sounding board or give you positive feedback. "Hey, I noticed you were out running earlier this week—good for you!" They can act as coaches, offering tips and honest, constructive criticism.

Of course, the reverse can be true as well—your social networks can sabotage healthy change by criticizing you or undermining your efforts. It's crucial to cultivate helpful, encouraging friends. Pursue conversations where you can get good information. Ask people in your network to support your efforts at healthy change and offer to be supportive in return.

2. Social networks influence your attitude.

We all tend to compare our own views with the views of those around us, and this is certainly true of attitudes toward body weight and other health-related issues. As I mentioned earlier, studies suggest that most people want to weigh a little less than the average in their social network; if the average goes up in your circle of friends and acquaintances, it's easy to follow suit and find your own weight creeping up. The opposite holds true as well. If the average weight in your network drops, you're more likely to lose pounds as the weight you find acceptable decreases. For this reason, it's important to seek out people who are living (and eating and exercising) the way you would like to live.

3. Social networks provide opportunities for engagement and attachment.

Engaging in social functions, church activities, group sports and recreation, or neighborhood functions can foster good feelings about yourself and your community and encourage healthy activity. Getting involved in activities around your neighborhood, for instance, spurs positive feelings about the area, which encourages people to get out and walk or play there. This, in turn, makes you and your neighbors feel more attached to your neighborhood. (Of course, social functions may also serve to undermine healthy living. We've all been to community or church events where the food is devastating to the waistline!)

WHAT IS YOUR SOCIAL NETWORK?

Most of us have never fully considered the make-up of our own social network. However, if you're attempting to make positive change in your life, knowing the nature of your network can make a huge difference to your success. To help you analyze your social network, here's a short social environment assessment, similar to the food and physical environment assessments you took earlier.

To start, do a quick inventory of your closest friends and colleagues and write down their names. Now think about the circles that you keep, including clubs, organizations, places of worship, etc., and write these down.

Next, keeping in mind these people and affiliations, fill out the quick assessment below:

YOU HAVE A CHOICE

Now that you have thought about your current social network, decide how you plan to move forward. If you believe that you need to change your network, there are three basic strategies:

- Approach 1: Adopt a new social network.

- Approach 2: Change the social network you're in.

- Approach 3: A combination of approaches 1 and 2.

As you contemplate making change, try to identify a social network that will bolster your efforts. This may be a network you already have in place, a whole new set of friends, or a blend of both. It may include individuals, organizations, and online networks. There is no single solution for everyone. You know yourself best. Tap into your knowledge of yourself to find a network that will best support you.

Social Environment Assessment

Social Environment			
FOOD	Positive	Neutral	Negative
	___Spouse or significant other supports healthy nutrition. ___Children are supportive. ___Most family gatherings include healthy foods. ___Friends are very supportive. ___Colleagues are very supportive. ___The organizations, clubs, or places of worship that I associate with are very supportive.	___Spouse or significant other is indifferent to healthy nutrition. ___Children are indifferent. ___Some family gatherings include healthy foods. ___Friends are indifferent. ___Colleagues are indifferent. ___The organizations, clubs, or places of worship that I associate with are indifferent.	___Spouse or significant other does not support healthy nutrition. ___Children are not supportive. ___Few, if any, family gatherings include healthy foods. ___Friends are not supportive. ___Colleagues are not supportive. ___The organizations, clubs, or places of worship that I associate with are not supportive.
PHYSICAL ACTIVITY	___Spouse or significant other supports an active lifestyle. ___There are exercise facilities at work. ___There are exercise classes offered a work. ___There are showers at work that I can use. ___There are parks or walking/running paths near work. ___ My employer pays for part of my fitness center membership.	___There are exercise facilities within a few blocks of work. ___I have access to parks or walking/running paths at work, but they are a few minutes away.	___There are no exercise facilities at work or nearby. ___There are no exercise classes offered at work. ___There are no showers at work that I can use. ___Work is not close to any parks or walking/running paths.
	Count up ✓:	Count up ✓:	Count up ✓:

In general, the more "positive" check marks you have, the more supportive your social network is of a healthy lifestyle.

What follows are suggestions for ways to think about changing your social network. These may trigger other ideas. Just be sure that what you do is aligned with your own preferences and values.

Face to face

A great example of the powerful benefit of face-to-face friendships comes from a woman named Michele, who recently wrote on our StrongWomen Facebook page. "I have been walking, then running, with the same 2 women for 15+ years now," she writes. "We try to go out Monday through Friday at 5:30 or 6 a.m., before work. One of the women has actually been driving from her home in the neighboring town to our neighborhood for all these days, weeks, months and years. There has to be a sense of commitment when somebody drives to your house. There's no rolling over in bed. Our morning sessions are an opportunity to get fresh air, observe nature, comment on current events, encourage, vent, motivate, and offer each other information and opinions about nutrition and exercise."

I'm partial to creating strong in-person social networks. As I wrote this book, I thought a lot about my own situation. Over the years, I've developed a strong network of family, friends, and colleagues who encourage my healthy lifestyle. My running partner, Steve, runs with me nearly every Saturday morning, and we rarely miss a weekend run together. Not only do we enjoy the runs themselves, but we love our weekly conversations: Over the years we've become a trusted resource for one another in our personal and professional lives. I also run with the Tufts Marathon Challenge team Wednesday and Sunday mornings. I know I wouldn't run three days a week if I didn't have Steve and the Tufts team there to encourage me. In addition, I rely on my family for company when I climb, hike, or ski.

When it comes to my food environment at home, my husband and I support each other in eating well. While he likes more chocolate and cookies around the house than I do, he usually stores these high up in a cabinet and not on the counter where they beckon to be eaten. (I do enjoy my cookies and a bit of chocolate—just not in the quantities he does!) Our kids, now mostly grown, also enjoy healthy eating, although they tend to snack too much on less-than-desirable stuff.

For many of us, our spouse or significant other and our children are our primary social network. Alas, they are not always supportive. On our StrongWomen Facebook page, Ruth wrote about her experience with this. "I've often felt undermined by my partner when trying to have better eating habits," she writes. "He tries to make me feel better with food and will 'treat' me when he knows I am trying to cut back. He means well but doesn't seem to understand that he's sabotaging me." In response, Milinda wrote, "My husband was identical! When I had to start losing weight to avoid knee replacement, he would constantly say 'Let's go out to eat' and then be upset because I said NO. With some people, it is their way of controlling us."

How to deal with unsupportive family members? Let them know that you really care about being healthy and that you need their backing. As we mentioned, most likely you're the gatekeeper of your house. The most important thing is to make changes slowly and deliberately over time. Be persistent. Give them some options. If you are cooking, let them know ahead of time that you are planning to cook a range of healthy meals. Which do they like best? Negotiate if necessary. Another tactic is stealth: Make just one change at a time, and do it so slowly that no one really notices!

I encourage you to seek out people within your current network of family, friends, and colleagues who will partner with you to create healthy change. Consider looking within your circles for a person or persons you respect and would like to emulate. Find ways to connect with them. It may turn out that they, too, are keen to have a partner with whom they can be active, talk about nutrition, even cook together. One supportive person may be all you need. (Martha Peterson is a great example of this; she and her sister provide abundant support for one another. At least once a week, they text each other with their respective body weights and how active they've been. They're both accountable to one another, supportive through thick and thin, and never critical.) Or you may surprise yourself and find a whole new set of friends for life. There is no magic number. The key is securing reliable social support for your efforts at healthy living.

Supportive organizations

As I mentioned, on most Wednesday and Sunday mornings I run with the Tufts Marathon Team. This team was started by our president at Tufts University, Larry Bacow. With two other close colleagues, we've supported the training of more than a thousand recreational runners to run in the Boston Marathon. Many people who ran with us six or seven years ago still come out to run, regardless of whether they're training for the marathon. I've made some wonderful new friends and colleagues this way. The first couple of years, I ran the race with the team (and may run one more time with my daughter), but in general, I no longer race. Instead, I enjoy the camaraderie of the team and relish my weekly runs with them.

Fortunately, there are hundreds of groups and organizations out there to support you. For some people, it's a formal organization such as Weight Watchers or programs at wellness centers. If these work for you, seek them out. For others, it's a club devoted to running, walking or cycling, or a fitness or community center. For still others, it's joining an organization that encourages outdoor activities, such as the Appalachian Mountain Club.

Our StrongWomen Program is a good example of a group that can provide abundant support (more about the program in Chapter 7). The program was developed to help women come together to exercise and eat well. Among its most potent benefits are the long-lasting friendships and social encouragement that come out of the classes. Sharon, a StrongWomen Program leader, recently commented, "My StrongWomen group of ladies is very supportive. They appreciate the time it takes to have this program. I support them with praise during the class and let them know they are doing an awesome job." Christine, another program leader, commented, "I have stopped advertising my Strong Women, Strong Bones program. Participants invite friends and make friends at the class. They are missed when they aren't there."

Exercise classes provide a natural supportive network. On our StrongWomen Facebook page, a woman named Susan wrote, "I attend a water aerobics class four mornings a week with a group of women, many of whom have been together for about 20 years. This group has had many joint replacements and realizes the importance of continuing with their water fitness. Plus, wonderful friendships have developed over these many years as we support each other through difficult times and good times. I am sure it is the closest group of friends that I have, as we also value our fitness efforts."

Faith-based organizations are increasingly providing support for nutrition and physical activity. A UCLA study recently surveyed faith and fitness in African-American women. The article reported that the women who participated in fitness groups that also included faith, such as listening to scripture readings or taking part in faith groups, participated in more fitness activities for longer periods of time. Across the country, there are more and more such programs. Congregations provide a natural network of people to help support healthy lifestyle efforts. I'm hopeful that the foods served at faith-group gatherings will shift toward more healthy options to further support good nutrition.

Volunteer groups are another option. This may sound off target, but in fact, volunteering in your community for projects related to physical activity or nutrition, such as cleaning up parks and playgrounds or bringing a farmer's market to town, helps to reinforce your own positive behaviors. You'll read more about this in Chapter 6.

Participating in a group of some kind almost inevitably results in opportunities for important new long-lasting friendships that will expand or reinforce the strength of your social network. When Deanne Hobba made the decision to shift her social network, she didn't abandon her old friends, but she did find a world of new friends by joining local running groups and races.

Online social networks

I recently started a StrongWomen Facebook page to provide women with social support and current information to enhance their health. I approached this with some skepticism, feeling that I had to research the idea extensively before launching the page. What I found is that online social networks such as Facebook can be used as highly effective tools for positive change, whether it's increasing voter turnout in the 2008 U.S. presidential election or promoting democracy in the Middle East. For the most part, our StrongWomen Facebook page has been met with overwhelming enthusiasm. Thousands of women are connecting through active dialogue and sharing of experiences, advice, and overall support. I realize that online social networks aren't for everyone, but for some they can be extremely helpful. (I hope you'll visit our site at Facebook.com/StrongWomenwithMiriamNelson; you don't have to be a member of Facebook to visit the site.)

The past few years has seen an explosion of online social networking and self-monitoring resources. In researching resources for this chapter, I came across numerous sites that provide tools and networking for nutrition, exercise, and weight control. Among them are weightcircles.com, weightlosswars.com, fatsecret.com, and extrapounds.com. You may find some benefit in these. No doubt, others will be launched in the near future. When evaluating a site, I encourage you to use your common sense. If what's promised sounds too good to be true, or if a site is touting (or selling) some strange nutrition, physical activity or weight loss advice, be wary.

Here are the three sites I felt warranted more thorough investigation (all of them are free):

Lose It!

What is it?

Lose It! is an iPhone application, but it can be used on the internet by individuals who do not have an iPhone or iPad. In general, it's intended to keep users organized and informed about what they're consuming each day and how many calories they're burning. When the application was introduced in

2008, more than 5 million people downloaded it to their phones. Lose It! emphasizes five pillars: Embrace mindful empowerment, track your calories, track your habits, track your exercise, and benefit from peer support. Lose It! was listed on the *Washington Post*'s 18 best iPhone applications in August of 2010. The Lose It! program has a Facebook page and a Twitter account.

How do you use it?

Lose It! functions as an online (or on-phone) food and exercise journal. You enter the foods you eat each day and the exercise in which you engage. The application gives you a budget of calories for the day based on your height and weight and on how much weight you would like to lose. To keep you accountable, you can share information with your friends, such as amount of weight you wish to lose, amount of time you exercise and how many calories you burn. In addition, you can share your progress on Facebook or Twitter, and keep data private or share with friends.

StickK.com

What is it?

According to its website, stickK's mission is this: To empower you to better your lifestyle and achieve your goals, whether it's losing weight, running a marathon, or quitting smoking. The website says, "We offer you the opportunity, through 'Commitment Contracts,' to show to yourself and others the value you put on achieving your goals."

StickK.com was created in 2007 by two Yale professors, Dean Karlan, a professor of economics, and Ian Ayres, a professor at the Yale Law School and author of *Super Crunchers:*

Why Thinking-By-Numbers is the New Way to be Smart and *Carrots and Sticks: Unlock the Power of Incentives to Get Things Done*, as well as Jordan Goldberg, then a student at the Yale School of Management. The concept is based on two principles of behavioral economics: 1. People don't always do what they claim they want to do, and 2. Incentives get people to do things.

How do you use it?

The site encourages you to set a goal and decide on when and how it will be achieved. Then you establish stakes for achieving it. This may take the form of a Commitment Contract that is legally binding, or a "bet" against yourself, which involves putting a certain amount of money on the line (by charging it to a credit card). If you don't reach your goal, stickK will send a set amount to a friend or family member, or a charity or anti-charity (a cause you dislike). So, for instance, if your goal is to lose 2 pounds per week and you put $20 per week on the line, each week that you fail to lose the 2 pounds, $20 will be sent to your selected recipient. Participants also have the opportunity to choose a referee to monitor their progress toward their goal. In addition, they may choose supporters from other stickK participants to act as the "cheering section" by writing encouraging messages on their journal page. The stickK approach depends on the honesty of the participant and/or the monitor.

StickK has established communities based on shared goals. If your goal pertains to health and lifestyle, for instance, you join a Health & Lifestyle community. Other communities include Diet & Healthy Eating, Education & Knowledge, Exercise & Fitness, Green Initiatives, and Money & Lifestyle. Each community has a forum and a section called Expert Word, which publishes articles of interest to that community, written by professionals.

Sparkpeople.com

What is it?

According to Business Week, Sparkpeople is the number-one weight loss and fitness website, with more than 9 million users. It offers nutrition, health, and fitness tools, support, and resources. The website boasts a weight loss program to help people transition to a healthier lifestyle and stop ineffective dieting. It features fitness trackers, meal plans, and a community of members and experts devoted to helping you maintain a healthy lifestyle. Sparkpeople coaches provide recommendations for those who want to lose or maintain their weight. Among the staff members are a registered dietitian, a master chef and healthy recipe developer, a certified running coach, and a healthy eating expert. Many of the experts are also community moderators.

How do you use it?

To get started, you sign up and choose a goal—either to lose weight or to maintain a healthy lifestyle without a weight loss goal. You provide your height, weight, age, and medical conditions. The website then provides you with a weight loss goal and/or nutrition and fitness goals. You can share your goals with other people, if you like. You can also join a team aimed at a common goal—or choose to join SparkAmerica, where the total minutes of physical activity are tallied for all of America. The Sparkpeople program tracks your nutrition, fitness, and weight. A phone application allows you to enter the foods you eat each day along with your fitness information, including daily activity, and then calculates the calories you burn during the day. The website features daily blogs, an exercise of the day, recipes, message boards, and a point system as a reward for completing specific activities. The points can earn you virtual prizes that you can share with other members.

SHAPING YOUR SUPPORTIVE SOCIAL NETWORK

Once you have completed the Social Network assessment above and have read the various options for creating online and other supportive networks, you can decide what support you need and how you're going to go about creating it. You know yourself best. Decide what will work for you.

Think about the following questions:

- Which family member(s) will be supportive?

- Which friend(s) can you count on to join your efforts?

- Are there any new organizations or clubs that you would like to join?

- Are there any online communities you can join to strengthen your network?

Below, write down your vision of an ideal social network for yourself. Make it as detailed as you like. Use it as a guide to get your started, and then update as you begin to develop your network over time.

Ideal Social Network

My Ideal Social Network
Who in my family can be supportive, and how:
Which of my existing friends can be supportive, and how:
Which of my existing colleagues can be supportive, and how:
Who is a person (or people) I know with a lifestyle I would like to lead:
How I plan to get to know them better:
Organizations or clubs I'd like to join:
Online social networking site I'd like to join:
Each week, I would like to share experiences with:
I will minimize negative influences in my social network the following ways:

MOVING OUTWARD

You're now an expert on changing your own personal environment, both social and physical. What's remarkable is that the changes you make will have a profound effect on those around you. The next thing you know, you'll be at the center of a new network, with others wanting to join your efforts.

This will have the effect of further supporting your own positive behaviors.

Once we've created change in our own lives, the next step is to foster the ripple effect, creating change in our communities and beyond. I strongly believe that we can use the tremendous influence of social networks for this sort of positive change, both in ourselves and in others. Networks have the power to do what we cannot do alone. Our challenge now is to get them working toward creating an environment in this country that makes healthy living easier for all of us.

Chapter 6. The Ripple Effect

When Deanne decided to transform her own life, to radically shift to a healthier way of being, her efforts had a strong impact on those around her. This is the benefit and the power of social networks. Whether we intend to or not, we have a profound influence on our family, friends, and colleagues.

As a result of Deanne's efforts and her success, her roommate—a woman with severe arthritis—started exercising and not only took off pounds, but greatly improved her overall health. (She had previously gotten around only with the help of a cane, but after beginning to exercise, she quickly reached the point where she could walk 2 or 3 miles at a time without one.) In addition, says Deanne, "a coworker of mine at the time began working out and lost more than 100 pounds." Two other coworkers joined Weight Watchers and each took off about 20 pounds. Deanne's mother began trying to walk regularly, and her father and his wife now walk and ride bikes.

"The whole family is thinking more about their dining habits and being smarter about what they eat and how they exercise," she says. But her biggest thrill was having her sister train to run a 5K. "This is a huge deal," says Deanne. Her sister had also been obese for her entire life. Gastric bypass surgery helped her lose weight, but she was still very depressed. "Somehow I convinced her to take a boot camp course," says Deanne, "figuring that if nothing else, for one hour two days a week she would not be able to think of anything else but getting through the camp. It turns out that she loved it! She decided she needed a new challenge in her life and decided a 5K was it. I can't wait to run/walk beside her as she reaches this new goal."

The ripple spreads. Deanne's sister's changes rubbed off on *her* family. "They all ride their bikes on weekends now," says Deanne, "and her husband has joined her for a few boot camp sessions. She has enrolled her daughter in a Healthy Kids program that encourages exercise and healthy eating habits. It's amazing the life changes people can make," Deanne remarks. "I'm so proud of her."

Deanne's own transformation and her impact on those around her are truly inspiring. She started with the need to do something for herself, to address her poor health, and her actions inspired positive change in those around her. This, in turn, made it easier for Deanne herself to maintain a healthy lifestyle.

In this way, individual change can blossom into societal change, which then has a beneficial impact on the individual. It's a wonderful upward spiral that anyone can create!

Now that you're an expert on changing your own environment, both the social and the physical, you can make additional changes, as Deanne did, not only to support your own healthy lifestyle, but to help others as well. You'll see that making just a few alterations in your life can affect those around you, just as Deanne's efforts to improve her own health powerfully influenced her best friend, her parents, her sister and her family, her colleagues at work.

It turns out that the ripple effect is most powerful at penetrating three layers of our social networks. This means that your friend, your friend's friend, and your friend's, friend's friends are most strongly influenced by how you live. When you do the math, you quickly see that by gathering a network around you, you can have a significant influence on hundreds, if not thousands, of people.

This chapter encourages you to be the larger change you want to see in the world—that is, to take action to create positive change in your community and beyond. It shouldn't be so hard for us to live healthfully. We need to collectively transform the greater food and physical activity environment so that making sound, healthy choices is easier for everyone in this country, young or old, male or female. If each of us works to create change, we'll not only help our own generation live healthier lives, but we'll also create an environment for our children that makes healthy living easier.

A good start is to consider what's most important to you. If something is personally relevant, you'll be more motivated to get involved. Ask yourself, "What does my community need? My workplace?" If you choose a cause for which there is already interest, the going is often easier. But I know plenty of women who have taken on a challenge they started from scratch. This is tough work, but it can be very rewarding if you start with small steps and build a team or coalition of engaged people to help you.

You need not start a national program or get legislation passed to have an influence. Even the simplest act can make a difference—especially if that simple act is repeated by millions of others. It's the collective effort that matters.

SIMPLE ACTS

Simple acts can lead to meaningful change by demonstrating that people are thinking differently, which leads to shifts in behavior. One small change generates others. This is what social change is all about.

Below is a list of simple acts that almost anyone can do to influence their community and beyond. They require minimal time and effort, but together they can begin to create necessary change. These are only suggestions; be creative, think up others. As you gain self-confidence in making change, you may find that you want to do more.

Create open dialogue with your family and friends

Among the most important actions you can take is to initiate an informed dialogue about an issue that concerns you. Informed conversations about good nutrition and physical activity with your family and people close to you can have a big impact. The give-and-take engages family and friends in the issues and helps to create a joint sense of responsibility for change. Share a meal or take a walk with a friend or a group of friends to discuss the problem. Just talking together, having a shared understanding of an issue, and then together coming up with a single action to address it is a powerful first step and will likely lead to systemic change. Women are good at capitalizing on their strong social bonds. These are a real advantage, and we should use them more.

Start with your immediate circle

Do the things that positively affect your family. Cook more. (This need not be tedious or overly involved. Master a few good recipes that are quick, nutritious, and delicious.) Turn off the TV. (In doing so, especially during dinnertime, you're influencing the health of your family.) Don't underestimate the positive impact these actions may have on your family, and by virtue of example, on the families around you.

Be picky in purchasing your foods

Vote with your pocketbook. In buying or not buying food items, you're influencing what companies produce in the future. When manufacturers see that people no longer want highly sweetened beverages, they will offer beverages with less sugar. When they see that 100-percent whole-grain breads are selling well, they will begin to develop new product lines featuring 100-percent whole grains. Consumers drive product development, so let's drive it in the right direction.

Be choosy about where you shop

What stores you patronize also matters. If you support businesses that sell the best produce and other healthy foods, these will prosper. This includes corner markets, mobile markets, local grocery stores, and farmers' markets.

Be an informed voter

Know where public officials stand on issues of agriculture, nutrition, and public health, and elect the officials who are most likely to champion sound legislation in these fields. The same goes for the school board, town mayor, statewide officials, and President of the United States. Vote for initiatives locally and statewide that foster good nutrition and physical activity.

Choose where you eat out

Wherever you live or travel, patronize the restaurants with the healthiest meals, including small portion sizes.

When you eat out, ask for healthier foods

Several years ago, when we were just beginning our community engagement work in Somerville, Massachusetts (see Chapter 8), we decided to try to influence the fare offered by restaurants. When Tufts undergraduate students visited local restaurants, we encouraged them to ask three questions: "Do you have brown rice instead of white? Do you have whole grain rolls instead of white rolls? May I have a larger portion of vegetables and a smaller portion of starch?" At least some of the restaurants responded in a positive way by offering brown rice, whole-grain rolls, and larger portions of vegetables. Supporting local restaurants and voicing your desire for healthy meals helps keep these restaurants moving in the right direction.

When you eat out, ask for calorie counts

New national legislation, part of the Health Reform Act, requires restaurants to provide consumers with menu ingredient labels, which include calorie counts. This information can help you choose healthier options. You may be surprised to learn that a salad may not be as healthy as a whole grain sandwich because of excess fat and sugar added to the salad dressing and toppings. Until ingredient labels are on every menu at every restaurant, ask for them.

Walkabout

When you go for a walk in your neighborhood or community, you're showing others that it's safe and fun to do so. You'll also begin to identify places in your community where there are dangerous crosswalks that need to be modified or where sidewalks or paths should be safely linked with a simple connector. Then you can address these issues with the leadership in your community.

Have active work meetings

For a brainstorming session or meeting, suggest to a colleague that you go for a walk instead of sitting at a conference table. You may even find that the ideas you come up with are more innovative.

Invite a neighbor to do a walking errand

Grab a neighbor and do an errand or two together once a week by walking—even something as simple as a trip to the corner store or to mail a letter at a post box. This way, you get the pleasure of socializing while accomplishing things on your to-do list.

Make a donation

Perhaps the simplest act of all is to make a donation to an organization dedicated to improving our nutrition and physical activity patterns. These organizations are diverse, ranging from local to national. Please see resources at the back of this book for a list of relevant and worthy organizations. Those of us with limited time can still make a huge difference just by offering financial support.

MORE ENGAGING ACTIONS

The suggestions below require a greater level of engagement. They take time and energy, but they can be highly rewarding and will help to turbocharge the movement.

Meet with community leadership

Wherever you live, your community leadership makes daily decisions that influence your health—decisions about transportation, restaurant and grocery store zoning, parks and recreation, schools, sidewalks, bike racks, etc. Meeting with leadership or speaking up at town meetings to advocate for public action that promotes health in your community fosters positive change. You might consider advocating for healthier meals at schools or for opening up school recreational grounds to community members. Many schoolyards across the nation are locked after hours, which means that their facilities can't be used for community recreation and physical activity. Advocating for safer sidewalks and bike lanes in your community is also critical for increasing active transport. There are movements afoot to change this, but they need support.

Serve on a community board

Many community and state boards have the potential to drive beneficial change by increasing access to healthy foods and physical activity. By joining one of these boards, you can help them make sound decisions and foster positive change.

Join an existing coalition

Many communities already have coalitions that need additional manpower. Explore your municipal website, talk to friends, and consider assisting a coalition that is focused on access to healthier food and/or increased physical activity.

Form a coalition

If you identify an issue with no advocacy group, you can form your own coalition—say, to provide farmers' markets in your neighborhood or to promote converting rails to trails in your community.

Gather friends for a regular walk or other exercise

For several years in a row, five of my neighbors came over to my house every Saturday morning to lift weights. It was a really fun and productive time. We caught up on the week's events as we got stronger together. All of the women are more active now than when we first started gathering. Walking, cycling, or lifting weights with friends can be a fantastic way to get fit and socialize at the same time. If you do this regularly, others will want to join or create their own groups.

If your children play sports, help to set a healthy snacking policy

A lot of unhealthy food is provided to children during and after sports. Work with other parents to develop a healthy snacking and beverage policy. For sports lasting less than an hour, there is no need for sugar-sweetened beverages (including sports drinks). Fruit and water are sufficient.

Help to clean up your local park

A safe, clean park is an ideal place for play, for children and adults alike. Organizing an annual or biannual clean-up day for a local park not only promotes the park (and the pleasure of playing there) but also helps to create a sense of community cohesion.

Write to elected officials

Write to your local, state, and national elected officials. One of my most interesting jobs was a one-year fellowship in the

U.S. Senate. I worked as a legislative assistant on health and human services for Senator Leahy, the senator of Vermont (my home state) and chair of the Agriculture, Nutrition, and Forestry Committee. From this work, I learned that constituents drive policy, and that writing campaigns work.

Write to encourage your elected officials to pass initiatives that promote access to healthier foods and physical activity of all kinds. For example, you might consider supporting the effort to have improved, easy-to-grasp labels listing calorie content and portion size on packaged foods and for restaurant meals. Or encourage local leaders to apply for a grant from the federal government's Let's Move initiative against childhood obesity. (The initiative is devoting $400 million in grants to bring grocery stores and farmers' markets to underserved communities.) Or push for the introduction of affordable transportation (e.g., bus or shuttle lines) to supermarkets or grocery stores currently located outside your communities. Or call for local leaders to improve their land use policies by encouraging the construction of parks or playgrounds and restricting further encroachment of unhealthy food venues into neighborhoods. Local governments can also promote the use of vacant land for community gardens or farmers' markets.

Better yet, run for elective office

By working as a public servant, you can have a profound influence on your schools, your community, and your state. At my StrongWomen summits, I ask women what they plan to do for themselves and what they plan to do for their families, communities, and beyond. One woman told me that she had never run for elected office, but she planned to do so over the next year. When she attended our next summit a year later, I was so pleased to hear that she had been elected to her community school board and was currently working to improve the foods served at local schools.

Grow produce in your yard

You need not convert your entire lawn to vegetables, but try growing some fresh vegetables, herbs, or fruit. Even a small patch—a tiny raised bed along your driveway or on your porch—will give you the delight of really fresh produce and will benefit your family and neighbors.

Help others plant a garden

Work in your community to open up space for neighborhood, school, or community vegetable gardens. Help your friends to plant a garden in their own yards. Encourage your local school to plant fruit trees. Schools are ideal sites for community gardens from which healthy fruits and vegetables can be harvested and sold cheaply to local residents. These gardens can be used to benefit children's education as they learn about basic plant biology as well as healthy eating and nutrition.

Support a local farmer

Local farmers provide us with fresh local food. To support their efforts, buy produce, meat, and cheese from them whenever you can. Encourage your friends to do so as well. Let them know that you value their work. You might even offer up a meal to them or volunteer to care for the farm for a brief period in the off-season so that the farming family can get some time away.

Write letters to the editor of your local paper

When community leaders are considering issues important to you, write a letter to your local paper to express your views. Encourage your friends to write in as well. Thoughtful letters influence community leaders.

Volunteer

Volunteering for boards and committees, serving (healthy) food at public events and leading trail walks all influence your local environment. Whether you volunteer one morning a week or one morning a year, your engagement will make an impact and also encourage others to get involved.

Influence the food and physical activity environment at work

Work with your colleagues to set policies on offering casual food in your office and on serving healthy food at meetings and celebrations. Put out that bowl of M&Ms on Fridays only. At celebratory functions, offer fresh fruit along with cake and cookies. For catered meals at work, have healthy options such as salads and vegetarian entrees, as well as sparkling water and fewer sugar-sweetened beverages. All of these strategies can help.

If your workplace has no exercise options at lunchtime, see if you can get your supervisors interested in offering exercise classes or adding a fitness program to your employee benefits. If your workplace doesn't have a shower, try to inspire interest in building one.

Commute by active transport

If more of us insist on commuting by active transport (walking, cycling, taking public transportation), our towns, cities, and transportation leaders will respond by making our roads safer and providing more transportation options.

All of the above are meaningful efforts that will help to improve nutrition and physical activity within your own life, your family, your community. To transform our larger environment, we need women from every walk of life to develop networks that engage in these sorts of efforts.

Recently, I saw a poster in the Geneva airport, home of the World Health Organization. It showed a beautiful photograph of an African woman, and the caption below her read, "Women: The world's greatest untapped resource." It's true. Women are a powerful force in the world. For one reason or another, we haven't tapped our full potential. We need more women moving together in a united front. We have our work cut out for us. Fortunately, an intriguing and ever-expanding group of inspiring women are leading the way and offering practical guidance on how to move from changing ourselves to changing our world.

Chapter 7. Game Changers

In my research at Tufts University, we've found that creating healthy change on a large scale requires engaging champions willing to serve at the local, state, and national level—and that much of the time, these champions are women. When it comes to social change, women are often the game changers. They see a need and rise to the occasion. Moreover, many women have an amazing ability to motivate others in their social networks to join their effort, or to nurture in others the desire to create their own change.

Two years ago, I decided to work with my colleague, Dr. Sara Folta, to study some of the women who have been highly successful at launching and leading programs focused on changing the way we eat and move in this country. We identified and interviewed sixteen women from around the country who have been driving forces behind exciting movements to create positive environmental change. The purpose of the study was to identify any shared strategies from which we might be able to learn. Here are the stories of a few of these women—what spurred them to action and how they achieved their goals. You've read about bits and pieces of their work throughout the book. Here are their full stories, which shed light on how we can move from transforming ourselves to transforming our world.

NEELAM SHARMA: COMMUNITY SERVICES UNLIMITED

Neelam Sharma wants people to eat healthy food. She also wants them to be able to find that good food in their own communities. For the past eight years, she has served as Executive Director for Community Services Unlimited Inc. (CSU), a nonprofit organization aimed at encouraging residents of her neighborhood in South Central L.A. to eat and grow their own food.

"You have to put healthy, affordable food where people have access to it," she explains. Sometimes that means persuading a supermarket chain to open a grocery store in a neighborhood; sometimes it means establishing a local farmers' market. Sometimes it means reclaiming unused urban space around your own community—lawns, driveways, empty lots—to grow your own food.

Neelam is a force in the local-food revolution. Her interest in creating local sources of healthy food grew out of her personal need to provide for her own family. In 1996, she moved to South Central L.A. with her young son and a newborn baby. Almost immediately, she experienced a kind of culture shock. She had grown up in England, where healthy food was more readily available, even in low-income communities. "My mother cooked every day," says Neelam. "She cooked real food, Indian food. I was very fortunate in that I never had to eat frozen dinners or anything. We ate real food, real salad every day."

When Neelam arrived in L.A., she was unhappy that she and her neighbors didn't have easy access to high-quality affordable food. "There was one farmers' market about 2 or 3 miles from where I lived," she recalls, "but outside of that, there wasn't much." She began to plant a few vegetables in her small backyard. "For the first time in my life, I began to seriously grow food and actually found that I was really good at it," she explains. She drew on memories of gardening with her father. "I also just kind of learned it out of books and by talking to other people," she says. To create more space for her garden, she pulled up her lawn and the concrete around her house. "Over a period of time, I essentially converted the entire front- and backyard into a community urban farm."

At the same time, Neelam became concerned about what her young son was eating in his local public school. She saw firsthand what she already suspected, that students were eating quantities of junk food. The L.A. district is the country's second largest school district, with more than 700,000 students at 885 schools. Ubiquitous in all the schools were sugary beverages, including sodas, which were readily available to the students in vending machines and student stores.

Neelam's first impulse was to network. "I have always been involved in some way or other with organizing around issues of social justice in whatever community I've lived in," she explains. She grew up in London during the late 1970s and over the years helped organize campaigns for the rights of immigrants living in her community.

When it came to the issue of food in the L.A. schools, Neelam knew what to do. She made contacts with like-minded parents and with students, teachers, and community members who shared her concerns. "We wondered if there was really anything we could do," she recalls. "We realized that we couldn't be effective focusing on change just in one school. We had to make a bigger effort." In 2001, she worked with others to found the Healthy School Food Coalition (HSFC), a group devoted to creating a new food environment in schools across the L.A. district.

"We met over the course of a year and looked at all of the legislation related to food in the schools," recalls Neelam. "We did a lot of homework." The first issue to tackle? Everyone agreed: Soda. "We were told by other people, 'Don't bother; you'll fail'," says Neelam. But we didn't listen; we launched a strong campaign, rooted in the school community and supported by parents, teachers, and students." Despite abundant community backing, the school board was opposed to the idea, with the exception of one member who offered barely lukewarm support.

"We kept at it, working together to persuade community leaders," says Neelam. Members of the HSFC each delivered to a school board member a quart-size Mason jar of refined sugar —representing the amount consumed each week by a typical teenager drinking two sodas a day. The group garnered grassroots support with email, letter-writing, and phone campaigns. Thanks to these efforts, the L.A. school district eventually unanimously passed a healthy beverage motion that came to be known as the "soda ban," effectively prohibiting the sale of sugary beverages in all L.A. schools. Sodas and other sugary drinks in vending machines, student stores and cafeterias were replaced with water and 100-percent juice, dairy and nondairy milk, and lower sugar sports drinks.

This was a major victory, but there was still a long way to go in changing the school food environment. Shortly thereafter, under pressure from Neelam's group and others, the L.A. school district enacted an Obesity Prevention Motion. The motion limited saturated fat, transfat, sugar, and sodium content for food sold in schools. It also set limits on portion sizes for snacks and sweets and boosted the variety of fruits and vegetables available at school lunches. Finally, it made the school cafeteria into a place of learning for students.

Neelam had seen firsthand that many students saw no connection between what they ate and their health. She believed that teaching kids by encouraging them to grow and taste local foods would have a greater impact on their desire to eat better than simply telling them that they should eat more fruits and vegetables. "You don't change people's eating habits by preaching to them," she says. "You do it by engaging them in very real activities that open their eyes to how food actually tastes."

One idea? To create an edible school yard, where students could taste local food they raised themselves. It would seem like an easy idea to promote, but Neelam and her colleagues at CSU faced an obstacle. They were denied a request for funding until they had conducted a "needs assessment" of the community first, to determine whether the program was really necessary. Neelam was undaunted. She and her group put their heads together to do a neighborhood food assessment. "We walked the community and mapped everything to do with food," Neelam explains. The project was completed over a nine-month period with the help of some 750 participants, including local middle-school and high-school student interns.

"The results were really eye opening," says Neelam. In an area one mile by 1.5 miles, for instance, they found only 8 restaurants, but 50 fast-food chains and 39 liquor/mini-markets. When participating community members were surveyed, 96 percent of respondents said they ate regularly at fast-food restaurants. But when asked what sort of food environment they wanted in their community, they ranked among their top choices a healthy supermarket, a farmers' market, and especially nutrition education. "What really struck me was that people know there's a health problem connected with how they're eating. But they're caught up in their lives, holding down jobs, and don't see a way out that's accessible to them. They had a really good vibe with what we were doing. They saw local kids conducting the assessment, and they said, 'Oh, good. Someone's doing something about this!'"

After the assessment was completed, Neelam took action. "It was not a grand plan, really. We started with three small plots at one elementary school around the corner from where I lived. Then we planted fruit trees to go with these," says Neelam. "Like so many things, it starts with a little idea that takes on a life of its own." Not long after, Neelam assembled a group of hundreds of parents, students, and teachers to plant massive tree orchards at two elementary schools, 75 fruit trees at each site: peaches, plums, nectarines, and varieties of apples you can't buy in stores. Later, they supplemented the orchards with orange and fig trees for more variety.

"We talked about the produce in our afterschool programs and offered tastings of whatever was in season," says Neelam. "This is the best way to teach about local foods. You can lecture kids, but it doesn't mean anything if you're not impacting their senses. Once kids taste something like a fresh local nectarine or apple, they can't believe it. It's a miracle every time. Their only experience has been apples shipped from far away —waxy fruit with no taste. When they taste a real apple or orange from fruit trees growing in the school yard, they're into it. With every new round of kids, it's the same; they end up lining up for second and third helpings of things they thought they wouldn't like—eggplant and collard greens. They feel a sense of ownership; they raised these vegetables themselves. They go home and tell their parents, begging them to buy fresh salads and oranges."

"This is what breaks my heart sometimes. Kids are so much more open to new ideas than adults are, open to the taste of new foods. You see kids trying to persuade their parents to buy local grapes for them."

To make it easier for families, Neelam organized farm stands at the elementary schools, so parents could grab fresh vegetables and fruit when they came to pick up their children. As a result of these educational initiatives, families in the community have started their own home gardens.

"The kids go home and talk about it, ask for seeds, and their parents come to us and ask, 'Can I get a fruit tree for my house?' So we established an annual fruit-tree giveaway. This is our fifth year. We give out 200 fruit trees a year, and they all go directly to the neighborhood. One woman stopped by the school recently to tell us she had a peach tree from us that had given her massive amounts of fruit. She wanted another tree. This is how it works: Things acquire a life of their own, they build exponentially.

"This is what keeps me motivated to do my work," says Neelam. "It's the changes I see in people, the changes I see in the environment—the fact that we now have affordable, really good-quality food in our neighborhood and people have access to it. This is great, seeing that local families can come and get their bags of fresh fruits and vegetables from our local produce stand. And seeing all the young people who are impacted by the programs in the schools and our training programs. One of our interns, for instance. Her mother came to her internship graduation last spring, and she asked, 'How do you do it?' She said that her daughter, age 16, now eats salad and vegetables, and that she would never have eaten these things in the past.

"To actually see the penny drop, to see people shift in terms of how they view food, how they suddenly see their own role in the world, in terms of not just having to be receivers of whatever is handed to them but being agents of change."

This is Neelam's measure of success: the brigade she leaves in her wake. "I will have been successful in this work when I am able to leave and other young people from the neighborhood are running the work."

To women interested in making a positive impact on healthy eating in their own communities, Neelam has this to say: "Look at where you live and see what changes need to be made. There are things that need to happen in every single community. Look at your own community and think about what needs to happen there."

When it comes to encouraging the growing and eating of healthy food, the type of change that's required may depend on the specific environment. L.A. is different from Chicago, as she points out. "But wherever women are, they can find a way to grow food somewhere," she says, "raising lettuce in a window box, for instance, or rustling up a bunch of neighbors to take over an empty lot, or finding space in a school. Growing food is a really important thing to do. Just one person raising food can have immeasurable effects on a neighborhood," she says. "People stop by to say, 'Hey what's that? Can I get a cutting or some seeds?' It's amazing what a tremendous impact you can have on people, and how the idea spreads."

Another way to make a difference is to build direct links with local farmers, says Neelam. "Of course, local has different meanings depending on location. But wherever you are, you can set up a collective buying program. This has two positive effects: It builds a market for local farmers and provides healthy food for people in the community.

"What gives me hope," says Neelam, "is that some of the crises we have created are fixable if we make up our minds to fix them. We can turn around a situation quickly—if we want to. All we need is a shift in our mindset."

BARBARA MCCANN: COMPLETE STREETS

It was the difficulties of a daily bike ride that drove Barbara McCann to launch a revolution—one that makes it possible for people to be more active in their everyday lives.

In the early 1990s, when Barbara was working as a writer and producer at CNN, she wanted to bicycle to and from work. "I was very aware of trying to be active on a daily basis," she says. Commuting by bike was a way of getting moderate physical activity and staying fit despite a demanding office job that required sitting for long periods of time. "It was a 'lazy' way to get exercise," she says. "It became a real health touchstone for me. I organized my life around it."

Biking in Atlanta wasn't easy. The streets were largely hostile to anything but cars—narrow, congested, and high-speed. An idea came to Barbara in a flash. "I was riding my bike on Ponce de Leon Avenue, and I had this thought, 'What if every street had a bike lane?' It was a sort of little vision ... that our transportation should be more multi-modal."

It was the birth of radical concept, one that might not only transform our streets and highways but also aid the fight against overweight and obesity. "America's roads are built mostly for high-speed movement of cars, making them dangerous and unpleasant, with few opportunities for physical activity," says Barbara. Why not make them safer and more agreeable for pedestrians and bicyclists?

In part because of this spark of insight on her daily bike ride to work, Barbara got interested in reporting for CNN on transportation issues. Among these was sprawl, an issue just coming to the attention of the public. "I realized this was not something that was only happening in Atlanta. This was really a nationwide issue. I started to do some reporting on it," she recalls. "Then I did a documentary and became more and more involved."

It was 1998, and Barbara realized that she was ready for a career switch. "I wanted to be less of the dispassionate journalist and make a more direct difference in the world." She got a job at a transportation advocacy organization. "It was a kind of 'go-to' organization" to answer questions everyday people would ask about transportation. Her *Mean Streets* reports looked at pedestrian safety and found that the risks of walking in automobile-dominated areas were driving pedestrians off the streets.

"Walking in the United States is a dangerous business," the report concluded. "Per mile traveled, pedestrians are 36 times more likely to die in a collision than drivers." The most dangerous places for walking tended to be in newer southern and western metropolitan areas, including Tampa, Atlanta, Miami, Orlando, Jacksonville, Phoenix, West Palm Beach, Memphis, Dallas, and New Orleans. In these cities and in many other places around the country, Barbara found, people are taking far fewer trips by foot because walking has become unsafe and inconvenient. Barbara feels this is especially true for women. "We tend to be sensitive to having a safe, comfortable environment in which to exercise; we tend to be more cautious about traffic issues. This means that a growing number of us are facing another type of danger," Barbara says, "the health conditions and diseases associated with a sedentary lifestyle. Human beings are supposed to be active," she adds; "it's our natural pattern. And it feels good to use the body on an everyday basis."

The risks of inactivity are well understood. But, as Barbara observes, it has taken some time for public health officials to realize that we're never going to get everyone to go to the gym. "People need to get exercise in their daily life," she says. "Walking to and from work and shopping is a natural way to build activity into the day. And research shows that moderate exercise, even in small spurts, has a big impact on health. So officials started to come to us in the transportation world and say, 'Gosh, can we do this work together?'"

Barbara participated in the first national study looking at links between a built environment and the health of people who live there. Called *Measuring the Health Effects of Sprawl,* the project was nicknamed by its authors "Sprawl makes you fat." "And indeed that is what we found," says Barbara. "Of course sprawl itself doesn't actually make you fat, but there is a relationship." People who live in sprawling areas are likely to have a higher body mass index and weigh six pounds more than people living in more compact areas. One reason? Because sprawl discourages walking and biking, robbing people of the health benefits of these and other kinds of physical activity that should be a part of everyday life. The report was published in the *American Journal of Preventive Medicine* in 2003, and it got a tremendous amount of media attention. "Something like 50 million Americans heard about it," Barbara recalls. "This launched discussion of the idea that the way we built communities contributed to people's ill health. Up until this point, no one had really talked about this in depth. This report put the issue out for public debate—and it has stayed there."

Now Barbara turned to addressing the problem. She began working part-time for an organization called America Bikes, advocating a bill that would reform federal transportation laws. "The idea was that every time we build a road, we need to think about accommodating bicyclists," she explains. "Believe it or not, there are eight national bike organizations, and they all worked together on the authorization of the federal bill." Unfortunately, the idea didn't sell well on Capitol Hill.

Barbara understood that the reform couldn't be just about bikes. Streets should cater to all users whenever possible; they should include sidewalks and crossing opportunities for pedestrians, bike lanes or wide paved shoulders, special bus lanes, and comfortable and accessible public transportation stops. "It's very strange to me that people tend to think of transit separate from road, separate from bike facilities, separate from pedestrians instead of thinking of it as a whole," says Barbara. "I've always had this more holistic view, and it has always been a driving force.

"I realized that we needed a new name for thinking about and talking about how to make the transportation system work for everybody." Barbara and her colleagues coined the term "Complete Streets" in 2003 and started the National Complete Streets Coalition. The idea was to bring together lots of different individuals and organizations who might otherwise have focused on local projects and harness their energy to create change on a policy level. "Complete Streets is about taking amorphous individual problems and seeing how we might come together to trigger a bigger solution. The coalition concentrated on working to get a bill into federal transportation law that would foster adaptation and design of streets for all users: pedestrians, bicyclists, motorists, and those riding public transportation.

For Barbara, a big obstacle was organizing the loose-knit coalition of groups and figuring how it was going to work. "At the beginning, my heart was in my throat all the time," she recalls. "I felt very unsure of myself in the realm of organizing and leading a coalition. I was mostly a journalist, you know. But I didn't let it scare me too much, and I just sort of figured it out, piece by piece. I was patient with it and asked a lot of people to help me, leaned on a lot of people, got advice from them. I think that was a good strategy.

"I didn't form an organization in the traditional sense," she explains. "It wasn't like I said, 'Okay, I am going to form the National Complete Streets Coalition and make this a national movement. Not at all. It was more like, 'Here's this cool vision, don't you want to be a part of it, too?' We wanted lots of people to feel ownership of the idea. That's very powerful. And it has worked really well. We hit a tipping point where a lot of people both inside the coalition and outside it were working toward the same goal."

Over the past couple of years, Complete Streets has won support from a variety of groups. The public health community and the Centers for Disease Control and Prevention endorse it as a strategy in the fight against obesity, and the American Academy of Pediatrics supports the approach as a safe way of allowing children to be active in daily life. Not long ago, First Lady Michelle Obama asked the National Governors Association, "If you're already paving a new road … why not add a sidewalk or a bike path, too?"

"Unfortunately, the federal transportation authorization bill is dead in the water now," laments Barbara. But the House of Representatives has in hand a draft bill that includes a Complete Streets provision, and Barbara is working for the same in the Senate. In addition, the Coalition has continued to work for Complete Streets policies at the state and local level. In 2009, 45 jurisdictions nationwide adopted the policies, including cities, counties, and regional governments.

Barbara sees her work as coordinating, collaborating, and delivering the message. She is a powerful communicator, a good writer and presenter who knows how to network and deliver information in a persuasive way. "I'm pretty good at talking to people where they are, understanding who the audience is, that they may know almost nothing about the complicated world of transportation research, reform, or advocacy. Complete Streets is super-simplistic. It's about speaking to ordinary people and getting back to a really basic value. "I have this very strong vision of how things could be. Getting other people to see it and embrace it has been very gratifying."

Barbara says that she learned critical lessons from her first mentor, a politically savvy person, who helped her develop a strategic sense about how to move things forward and how to build relationships, "the right kind of relationships," as she explains.

"The way to make change isn't necessarily to completely redefine the universe, an ideal version of what you want to see," says Barbara. "It's more about seeing where we are now and then figuring out what leverage points you can push to make changes."

Barbara's focus has been on developing a network of relationships and figuring out projects to work on with the coalition's member organizations, including the AARP and the America Planning Association. "The collaborative approach has helped the coalition leverage lots of different people's expertise," Barbara says, "and that has been behind our overall success." To spread the word, she conducts Complete Streets workshops, working with planners, engineers, and other members of a community. "We spend a whole day with them talking about how to do Complete Streets. It's often very gratifying to see people get really engaged, really quickly. I can see their eyes kind of opening and their perspectives shifting as the day goes by."

Whole communities have benefited from the work of the Coalition. "The places that have been adopting these policies and then implementing them are doing very cool things on the streetscape," Barbara explains. "People who are walking and biking and taking transit have a safer place to do it. A good example is Charlotte, North Carolina. It's a pretty suburban kind of sprawling place. But they have really started to systematically go back and fix their road system and they've improved a whole bunch of intersections and put in a ton of bike lanes. They're experimenting with some innovative things such as road diets."

A road diet is just what it sounds like: making a road that's fat with multiple lanes thinner, safer, and more efficient. This means reducing the number of lanes and converting the extra space into bike lanes, walkways, median strips and parking. Road diets make streets safer for bicyclists and pedestrians and discourage speeding. "They have been shown to reduce crashes by 18 to 47 percent," Barbara notes. "They can be done with simple paint. And they look great. The Complete Streets of Charlotte are gorgeous. There are examples like this all over the country."

"There's a very specific reason for women to work toward Complete Streets," says Barbara. "Women are the bus drivers of our society, ferrying kids around. If we can make our streets safer and more agreeable for walking and biking, this will make our kids more independent, able to move themselves."

For women interested in boosting physical activity by making the streets in their communities more livable, vibrant, and "complete," Barbara suggests getting involved on both the local and federal level. She believes that we are at a tipping point on this issue. More and more cities and counties are adopting Complete Streets policy, and there is support in the federal government. She encourages women to take a look at the landscape in their communities to see where the problems may be. "Then pay attention to who potential champions are in your community—who will be open to this in your city, county, and state planning organizations—and let them know how you feel," she says. "Being clear about what we want out of our street environment is important. Transportation officials are ready to hear it. We citizens can work with them toward a goal that's bigger than just moving traffic. But we need ordinary people talking about what they want and what they need."

JILL VIALET: PLAYWORKS

In 1996, Jill Vialet was waiting to meet with a principal from an elementary school in Oakland, California, a school that served a low-income population. "She was running late," Vialet recalls. "She came marching out of her office with that kind of aggravated, worked-up expression that only an elementary school principal can fully muster. She had these three little boys trailing behind her. She dismissed them to the secretary and then started in on a tirade about the litany of reasons that recess was hell. How the teachers found every reason under the sun not to be outside at recess. How the kids didn't know the rules to games. How the same three little boys got in trouble every day, and how they weren't bad kids, but they were starting to believe that they were bad kids. She was going on and on, and she finally kind of came up for air, took a deep breath, and looked at me and said, 'Can't you do something?'"

Jill was taken aback at first, but then realized that the principal's clarion call struck a chord with her. Recess wasn't like it used to be, intense play with a sense of boundaries, where everyone understood the rules of the games. Jill decided to try to help rebuild the culture of play, to make sure that kids knew the rules and had some basic conflict resolution skills. Within the year she had founded Sports4Kids, now known as Playworks, an organization devoted to increasing physical activity for kids in low-income and major urban areas by creating opportunities for safe, healthy, meaningful play. The organization sends trained coaches to hundreds of low-income, urban schools, where they transform recess and play into a positive experience. It also offers training and technical support to schools, districts and communities that want to bring safe physical play to children.

"I have this vision that one day every kid in America will get to play, every day," she says. "I'm pretty myopic about this." Jill thinks that a good leader should be a little myopic, to stay focused on the endpoint of her vision. For her, success is about "really sharing this vision in a way that is actionable and inspiring—and getting out of the way for a lot of other people who own the vision." Her organization employs a diverse corps of young adults fresh out of college to work with schools and "change the world through kickball." "They work so hard and are so playful and irreverent, and they care so much," says Jill. "Creating the opportunities for those young adults to really be part of the change is very sustaining."

Jill has been phenomenally successful in realizing her vision. Playworks is currently in 250 schools across 15 different cities in 10 states including Washington, D.C., affecting more than 100,000 students every day.

Jill credits her success to her sense of humor and her persistence. "I'm a salesperson trapped in a do-gooder's body," she says with a laugh. "My kind of M.O. is persuasion; my default mode is to sell. I think that's really contributed to my success. And I'm persistent, always trying to figure out if something is a 'no,' how to make it be a 'yes.'"

If you want to make change, Jill says, determine your strengths and play to these. When she talks to social entrepreneurs, she likes to tell a story about when she was in high school and her basketball coach made a simple point to her: If you just bend your knees, you can be better at any sport you play. Jill finds this an apt analogy for her belief in the importance of positioning yourself so that you can best use your own strengths, whatever your cause. "The first and most obvious thing about bending your knees is that you're in this ready position," she says. "You can respond really quickly. The position compels you to lead with the strongest part of your body as your first reaction. Especially as a woman athlete, my upper body strength is not great. So whenever I try and muscle through with my upper body, I'm never going to be as effective as I am if I use my legs first." So, says Jill, setting yourself up so that you can lead with your strengths and build a team around you of people who complement them goes a long way in building an organization that's effective and sustainable.

Jill finds that people are generally eager to help. "I get a kick out of how much people want to have meaning in their lives and how incredibly appreciative they are when they're given the opportunity to be a part of something bigger than them-selves."

CARLA MARCUS: WINTERKIDS

It isn't always easy to be active on cold winter days. And in a northern state such as Maine, where winter is the longest season, this can mean months on a couch, with little activity and a high risk of weight gain.

Carla Marcus understands this. She grew up in Maine, where a third of residents are obese. "Everyone you talk to will tell you, 'Oh, I'm such an active person, I swim in the lake and I bicycle and I play tennis.' But when you ask, 'What do you do in the winter?' they say, 'Oh, I hunker down and sit on the couch. It's true I gain a few pounds, but I'm so glad when the snow melts.'"

When Carla was growing up, winter always included plenty of skiing and other outdoor activities. In her view, there was a clear practical solution to the obesity problem in her state: get people moving year-round, especially children. In 1997, she launched a program to provide fifth-graders in Maine with access to winter sports, offering them a "passport" for free skiing at ski areas across the state.

Around the same time, she began hearing news of the statistics on childhood obesity and increasing cases of type 2 diabetes in children, which bolstered her passion. "I kept collecting more and more information, talking to doctors, pediatricians, family practitioners, getting anecdotal information from principals, teachers, and parents." She saw the downward trend in physical fitness in Maine, especially in winter, and recognized the opportunity to help children and families. Over the next few years, Carla's vision grew into WinterKids, an organization that helps children in preschool through twelfth grade across the state develop a lifelong habit of outdoor winter activity. The programs encourage skiing, snowshoeing, ice skating, tobogganing, dog sledding, and other winter activities.

"I wanted to get every kid and every family active outside in the winter. Though my interest is in health for the whole family, I focused on children because I know that children grow up to be adults. I also know that if you reach a child, you reach the family."

One story in particular brings this to light. After Carla started her fifth-grade passport program, she got a call from a Maine resident named Alicia who said, "I just want to tell you that you've changed our lives." Alicia's son Zach, a fifth grader, was highly asthmatic. He missed a lot of school because of his asthma attacks, and he had an especially hard time in cold weather. The drugs he was taking weren't working to reduce the severity of his asthma. But he wanted one of Carla's passports for skiing. Once he got one, he begged and begged his parents to let him use it just for one day, at a little local mountain close by. They gave in and said, "Okay, we'll both go with you." Within a year, Zach and his family had skied at 12 of the

13 mountains on the pass. Zach dramatically reduced his medicine—an improvement his doctor attributed to the Winter-Kids program.

As WinterKids expanded, Carla poured her energy into fundraising so that she could provide the programs for free. "Every single year we had more and more kids involved, more and more families participating." When Portland, Maine, was designated a center for resettlement for refugees from Somalia, Carla created an extensive new program to address the needs of the Somali community, for whom the winter climate was a brand new, threatening challenge. By the time Carla left WinterKids in 2007, some 30,000 residents of Maine were participating in the program.

Carla's success had a ripple effect across the country. "It became a national program, an outdoor learning curriculum. People were either replicating it or using our materials all across the country, so the numbers just continued to increase." She attributes her success to her ability to make things happen. "My strength is getting things done. I don't procrastinate. And I don't take 'no' for an answer."

"There really is very, very little that can't be done," says Carla. "Figure out where you want to go first, and then the steps that you need to make will fall into place. What do you want this program to achieve? What is its purpose?" Once you've established your goal, says Carla, then you need to garner resources: people, supporters, finances. "If you're trying to make anything happen, you need people to help you. You have to make them feel good about what they're doing. Stewarding supporters of all kinds is terribly important. But it's really just a matter of doing it. I don't want to sound like a Nike commercial, but that's really what it is, just do it."

STRONG WOMEN: ACROSS THE NATION

Neelam, Barbara, Jill, and Carla all had moments in their lives when they saw a need and were compelled to act. Neelam saw that there was no fresh produce available in her neighborhood. Barbara experienced the hazards of cycling to work. Jill observed that rambunctious schoolchildren needed a safe outlet for their energy. Carla understood that families living in northern climates lacked an easy way to be active during the cold winter months. Each of these women took a look at their surroundings and perceived a need for change, then rose to action. The movements they launched have changed the lives of thousands. But they often began with something simple, a moment of revelation or a small event that triggered their awareness.

I had a similar moment, a phone call that spurred me to start the StrongWomen movement.

If you had told me 25 years ago that I would be involved in a movement that would affect thousands of women, from Pratt County, Kansas, to Nome, Alaska, from Mt. Ida, Arkansas, to Lancaster, Pennsylvania, I would have said, "Not likely."

When I began my research career, I didn't set out to change lives. I just knew that I loved research and that I wanted to help people, to make the world a little better. I wanted to work with committed colleagues who wanted their research to benefit others. What I didn't know was what form that benefit would take. Or how many people would help me along the twists and turns of my path. Or how my vision would be sometimes fuzzy and sometimes clear. Or how serendipitous the process of launching change can be. It can start with a little wave that spreads quickly ... and not always in the way you anticipate.

Here's my story. Right after I married and had my first child, we moved to Boston. I had just finished a public policy fellowship at the U.S. Senate with Senator Leahy from Vermont. While I really enjoyed working in Washington, D.C., I missed research and wanted to return to Tufts, where I had earned a doctorate. The year was 1989.

With my mentor at the time, Bill Evans, and others, I helped to write a grant to the National Institutes of Health for a research project examining how strength training might affect bone density and risk factors for osteoporosis for women in midlife and older. It was a long shot, but we were fortunate. With collaborators from Columbia University, we received the funding and the go-head to work on the project. I didn't know it at the time, but this was the study that would launch my StrongWomen initiative.

The year-long study looked at postmenopausal sedentary women aged 50 and older. Half of the women continued their normal pattern of sedentary living; the other half came to our center two days a week and participated in a progressive strength-training program. Over the year, the ladies who were sedentary lost strength. They lost lean tissue and gained body fat. Their bone density decreased and they became even more sedentary. By contrast, the group that strength-trained became very strong, gained muscle and lost body fat. Their balance improved, as did their bone density at the hip and spine. They were more active in their everyday lives. Biologically, the women from the strength-training group were about ten to fifteen years younger than the women in the control group. These women reported that they felt more confident and took on physical challenges they had never thought possible, even at a younger age.

This was the first study to show that women in midlife and older could strength train at a high intensity and become more youthful over time. The prestigious *Journal of the American Medical Association* accepted our paper for publication. Soon after, I worked with Sarah Wernick to write a book to help women across the country benefit from the results of the research. We wrote a proposal, identified an agent, found a publisher, and less than two years later, *Strong Women Stay Young* was published. Much to my surprise and delight, the book became a *New York Times* bestseller. I was thrilled that the message struck a chord with so many women.

About a year later, I had my pivotal moment: I got a call out of the blue from a woman named Linda Tannehill. Linda was a cooperative extension agent in Kenai, Alaska, who ran community health programs as part of her job. She said that she found my book very helpful and that she was using it as a basis for community programs for women in her area. She and another cooperative extension agent she knew, Jean Clarkson-Frisbee from Kansas, asked me to develop the StrongWomen Program. That call triggered a decade of community engagement that has influenced the lives of thousands of women across the country who have led or participated in our programs.

The StrongWomen Program has far exceeded my expectations. With a network of StrongWomen ambassadors from eight states, we have trained more than 2300 leaders. The curriculum is now led in 35 states, including eight with large statewide programs: Pennsylvania, Arkansas, Kansas, Alaska, Colorado, Montana, Wisconsin, and Missouri. This is in large part because several very dedicated women recognized its potential and prodded me to make it a reality. Colleagues at

Tufts helped me create it, most notably Rebecca Seguin, and more recently, Sara Folta and Eleanor Heidkamp-Young. Most important, local community leaders who are on the front line running the programs have made it a wide-ranging success, changing the lives of women throughout their states.

States with StongWomen Programs

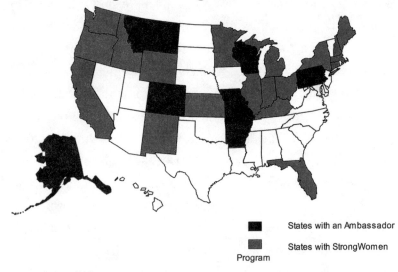

States with an Ambassador

States with StrongWomen Program

Our StrongWomen Program is now present in many states across the country, with ambassadors in seven states: Alaska, Arkansas, Colorado, Missouri, Montana, Pennsylvania, and Wisconsin. We also have a very strong program in Kansas. Since 2004, we have trained more than 2,300 program leaders.

The weekend before I wrote this section of the book, I was in Portland, Maine, to conduct a StrongWomen Healthy Hearts workshop with my colleagues. We were training 97 extension educators from 30 states to lead programs in their communities. These are wonderful women (and a few good men) who are dedicated to their work and the people in their community. The training not only gives them the tools they need to start their own community programs, but also helps them go through their own personal transformations. When they are inspired to improve their own lives, they are more motivated to change the lives of others. These program leaders empower the women who participate in their programs to eat more nutritiously and to be more physically active. These women, in turn, change the lives of others: family members, friends, colleagues. With this powerful network of women, our vision is beginning to be realized: To create a diverse community of women who are fit, strong, and healthy, and who are, in turn, agents of change for their families, communities, and beyond. Each success is a huge victory, but this is just one small road toward an ambitious goal.

Several times, as I looked out at the extension educators, I got choked up. I had so many women to thank for making this happen. The initiative may have started with that phone call, but then an army of wonderful, strong women and a few good men helped to carry it out.

Why do I think that the StrongWomen Program has been so successful? My collaborators and our key program supporters have made the biggest difference. But I also believe the program has succeeded because it is based on solid evidence that grows out of our ongoing research at Tufts University.

The weekend before I wrote this section of the book, I was in Portland, Maine, to conduct a StrongWomen Healthy Hearts workshop with my colleagues. We were training 97 extension educators from 30 states to lead programs in their communities. These are wonderful women (and a few good men) who are dedicated to their work and the people in their community. The training not only gives them the tools they need to start their own community programs, but also helps them go through their own personal transformations. When they are inspired to improve their own lives, they are more motivated to change the lives of others. These program leaders empower the women who participate in their programs to eat more nutritiously and to be more physically active. These women, in turn, change the lives of others: family members, friends, colleagues. With this powerful network of women, our vision is beginning to be realized: To create a diverse community of women who are fit, strong, and healthy, and who are, in turn, agents of change for their families, communities, and beyond. Each success is a huge victory, but this is just one small road toward an ambitious goal.

Several times, as I looked out at the extension educators, I got choked up. I had so many women to thank for making this happen. It may have started with that phone call, but then an army of wonderful, strong women and a few good men helped to carry it out.

Why do I think that the StrongWomen Program has been so successful? My collaborators and our key program supporters have made the biggest difference. But I also believe the program has succeeded because it is based on solid evidence that grows out of our ongoing research at Tufts University.

LESSONS LEARNED

What have I learned from my own experience, and from the efforts of Neelam, Barbara, Jill, Carla, and the other twelve women we interviewed? When I reflect on these shared experiences, I see that there are several keys to success:

See a need and seek a network of support

First and foremost: All of the women we interviewed saw a need in their surroundings and were compelled to do something about it. They were not willing to let the status quo stand. They saw the need, rose to the occasion, and networked to find support. As Neelam said, "Look at where you live and see what changes need to be made. There are things that need to happen in every single community. Look at your own community and think about what needs to happen there." Then seek like-minded people who can offer support.

Despite no clear road map, move forward anyway

Each of these women could envision the change she wanted to bring about, but none of them knew instantly how to achieve it. Each could see the big picture, but most were unsure how to proceed. Instead of getting bogged down in the details, they just moved forward in small steps. Over time, they became more strategic and deliberate. This meant that they had to take some risks along the way. As Barbara said, "The way to make change isn't necessarily to completely redefine the universe . . . It's more about seeing where we are now and then figuring out what leverage points you can push to make changes."

Seek help from others

I think that Barbara said it best: "I was patient with it and asked a lot of people to help me, leaned on a lot of people, got advice from them. I think that was a good strategy." This same strategy has made our StrongWomen Program so successful. I may have started things off, but success depended on the input and advice from my colleagues at Tufts, our extension educators, and thousands of local champions around the country. Find helpers who complement your skills. As Neelam put it, "One of my biggest strengths is knowing what my own weaknesses are ... and finding staff who make up for the things I am lacking." "If you're trying to make anything happen, you need people to help you," advises Carla. "You have to make them feel good about what they're doing." I couldn't agree more.

Stick to it

All of these women had an ability to keep going even when things got tough. Carla said, "My strength is getting things done. I don't procrastinate. And I don't take 'no' for an answer." Jill concurs: "I'm persistent, always trying to figure out, if something is a 'no,' how to make it be a 'yes'." This often means being adaptable. Ideas that are good at the start might need to be reevaluated and revised. Obstacles might seem insurmountable and setbacks, frustrating. But all of the women agreed: The important thing is to keep going.

Find guides and mentors

Barbara says that she learned important lessons from her politically savvy mentor. He helped her develop a strategic sense about how to move things forward and how to build relationships, "the right kind of relationships." Many different people have also guided my work. These mentors and models have been formal and informal. Seek out people who can offer advice or act as a sounding board. This is critical for moving ideas forward.

Have an ego but don't let it be the reason for your work

These women did not let their egos get in the way of their vision. Their work was not about them personally; it was about the collective effort to create change. I think that efforts can get foiled quickly if the person leading the change feels she must get exclusive credit. I'm not saying that it isn't important to recognize those who lead the way—just that recognition shouldn't be the driving force behind the work. All of these women were compelled to do their work because they believed it was the right thing to do. The important thing, said Jill, is "really sharing this vision. And getting out of the way so that other people can own the vision, act on it, and inspire others. "

Most important, do something that resonates with you and lead from the heart

As Neelam said, "My own need to provide for my family, for my children, led to the bigger piece of work I'm involved in. The question of how to access good food at home became: How do you affect these issues on a community-wide level? How you do you inspire and engage others to become involved in a cause? Think from the heart."

What struck me in this research were the similar strategies used by all of these women. Because their personalities and life experiences were quite diverse, we had expected greater diversity in approach. Some of the women were extroverts; others, introverts. Some were young; some older. Some were single; others had families. But it wasn't their personalities or life circumstances that dictated how they moved forward with their work. When it came to tackling social issues, a common approach guided them all: acting when you see a need, building a network of supportive people, moving forward regardless of a plan, persevering, and—most important—leading from the heart.

I find these life lessons deeply inspiring, useful in guiding us not only in our endeavors related to civic engagement, but also in life.

Chapter 8. Going Viral

What will it take to really turn things around in this country? It's going to take launching an epidemic of positive change and "going viral" with healthy transformation. It's going to take many people like Deanne and Martha, doing something for themselves, something difficult, in order to create positive change in their own lives—thereby deeply influencing the lives of those around them. For many women, this is the best possible way to make an impact. Others may wish to go further, as Neelam, Barbara, Carla, and Jill did, to create movements large or small, aimed at reshaping our environment on a local, regional, or national scale. The big change we need in this country will take both approaches and an army of us, engaged in all ways.

I'm optimistic that the time is right for this kind of radical transformation. It's an exhilarating moment. We're experiencing a groundswell of interest in how we eat and how we move. People are distressed by the high rates of obesity and inactivity. They're fed up (literally) with the scarcity of healthy food and the abundance of unhealthy food. While efforts to confront our weight issues have played out mostly on the personal level, there are exciting new movements afoot to address the larger, "obesigenic environment" piece of the problem. There's a gathering sense that our food system as a whole needs repair. Consensus is building about the importance of creating environments that promote physical activity.

There is political will to make change, both locally and nationally. First Lady Michelle Obama's *Let's Move!* campaign is a great example of this. Several companies in the food industry are realizing the need for a shift, and many of them are acting on it. Cereal manufacturers, for instance, are slowly reducing added sugars in their cereals—a small step, but a sign of the times.

At the community level, women such as Neelam are finding ways to bring fresh fruits and vegetables not only to their own backyards but also to the other residents of their city environments. In cities across the nation, women are promoting the creation of networks of sidewalks and bike lanes that help people on foot and bicycle get where they are going safely, just as Barbara did. Hundreds of other initiatives locally and nationally are beginning to gain traction.

These collective signs from various segments of society point toward an opportunity for a real shift—a tip toward meaningful social change that can spread virally.

ELEMENTS OF SUCCESSFUL SOCIAL CHANGE

At Tufts University we have examined the elements of successful social change on a large scale. My close colleague, Dr. Christina Economos, has led the effort. Several years ago, Chris asked the question, "Why have rates of breastfeeding, seatbelt use, recycling participation, and tobacco control improved? How did these movements get started and, more important, how did they get traction?"

With colleagues from around the country, Chris set out to answer these questions. She and others did a systematic evaluation of successful social change movements. They interviewed key individuals involved in each of the movements; they conducted thorough literature reviews, examined related policy changes and government regulation, analyzed the impact of the media, searched for the spark that launched the movements, and identified the major stakeholders who funded the initiatives. After two years of research, several themes emerged. Among the important shared elements that fueled the changes were the following:

A crisis—a precipitating event that pushed the movement to the tipping point. For recycling, it was the Long Island garbage barge incident in 1987. For tobacco control, it was the 1986 Surgeon General's report on the deleterious effects of secondhand smoke. After these events, the respective movements took off.

Science base. Having credible scientific evidence that a problem exists and that it has an impact on our well-being is critical for any movement. It wasn't until evidence came to light on the negative impact of formula-feeding on newborns' immune systems, intellect, and overall health that breast-feeding rates increased. Similarly, mounting evidence on the harmful effects of secondhand smoke motivated nonsmokers to advocate for change.

Economic impact. A problem gets the attention of state and national governments, employers, and citizens when it's clear that it carries significant costs—and when a solution clearly saves money. The use of seatbelts saved the nation $3 billion annually. When recycling began to cut costs, it gained steam.

The health care costs of smoking spurred large-scale policies aimed at reducing smoking rates.

Spark plugs. For nearly all of these social movements, there was a key individual or small group of individuals who sparked the change. For tobacco control, that was C. Everett Koop, Surgeon General at the time, and David Kessler, then of the Food and Drug Administration. For breastfeeding, it was Dr. Ruth Lawrence of the University of Rochester and Dr. Audrey Naylor of Wellstart International, among others.

Grassroots coalitions and advocacy. Coalitions help individuals with a shared vision and common objectives succeed. All of these movements were driven by multiple local, state, and national coalitions. Sometimes their efforts were coordinated; other times, not. What was important was (and is) the collective action and visible advocacy on the respective issues.

Government involvement. While it's clear that government cannot solve our social problems, it does play a crucial role. At the local, state, and national level, legislation that resulted in policy changes has had a major impact on generating shifts. Policies creating smoke-free public buildings and mandatory bottle recycling, for instance, helped the tobacco control and recycling movements gain traction.

Mass communications. Mass media influences society's attitudes, beliefs, and values. All of these movements used multiple media channels to communicate consistent and engaging messages, backed by solid scientific evidence.

Systems change. For many of the movements, a change in the system was also key. Take, for example, seatbelts. Prior to policy changes, seatbelts were clumsy and hard to use. After the changes, car companies developed new designs that made seatbelts more comfortable and easier to use. Having more local programs that made recycling easier and cheaper than not doing so reinforced recycling behaviors.

A plan. None of these movements had a single strategic plan. But as they gained momentum, they all made efforts to unify the various supporting groups and coalitions around a strategic, large-scale plan, one that engaged citizens and the media and drew community, business, and government support to work toward a common goal.

PUTTING THE STRATEGIES TO WORK

Since Chris's paper on the elements of successful social change movements was published in 2001, it has informed all of the research and public health programming in our research center at Tufts University. One of the most significant initiatives that grew out of this research was a program that started a year later, called Shape Up Somerville: Eat Smart. Play Hard.

Somerville is an urban community just north of Boston with a very diverse population and a significant childhood obesity epidemic. (At the time, 43 percent of children in Somerville were either overweight or obese by the time they reached fourth grade.) Chris thought that if we put together elements from previous successful social change movements and engaged the community to take the lead, we might literally reshape the entire community of Somerville. And with community engagement, that is what we did.

Working on Shape Up Somerville with Chris and other Tufts colleagues, as well as local leaders, has been one of the most rewarding experiences in my professional life. With federal grant support from the Centers for Disease Control and Prevention, we launched the program in 2002. We networked with myriad individuals and organizations within Somerville, at first to build awareness and to understand their needs, and then to create change in almost every part of their community.

Critical to the success of the program was the engagement of a powerful network of people living and working in Somerville. They took on the initiative as their own: Schools got involved, as did parks and recreation services, restaurants, children, parents, the local news media, health care professionals, and various coalitions.

To see if this "local" social change movement would actually translate into meaningful improvements in the health of Somerville's children, we monitored them over time. The results were powerful. After only one school year, the Somerville students were gaining less weight than the children in two "control" communities we were monitoring. The Somerville kids were still gaining the normal amount of weight they should gain as growing children, but they weren't putting on excessive weight. This was very exciting. In the end, it was many small changes that made the difference: menu changes at schools, cleaner parks, crosswalks at busy intersections, placards promoting healthier foods in restaurants, articles in the local newspaper, collective dialogue among parents and children, and a lot of other small, but important shifts in the community. Collectively, these small changes added up to real, measurable change.

Shape Up Somerville is now considered a model program for the nation. First Lady Michelle Obama highlighted it at the launch of her *Let's Move!* campaign, where the mayor of Somerville, Joe Curtatone, was on hand. Mayor Curatone has become a national leader in childhood obesity prevention, working to help town leaders throughout the nation understand that a healthy community is a strong community. The best news is that now, almost a decade after it started, Shape Up Somerville is still going strong and making a difference in people's lives.

I learned a lot from this project. I learned that people networking together can make real, enduring change; that in order to create this sort of sustainable change on the obesity issue, we need to address it at a large scale, at the community level and beyond; that many small shifts can add up. I learned that leadership matters. And I learned that social networks are immensely powerful in driving positive change. If it's true that our sphere of influence is three degrees, and only six degrees gets us to everyone in the world, then theoretically, at least, each of us has the potential to affect in some way, however small, nearly half the population of the world.

For this reason, I'm optimistic that meaningful and lasting change in how we eat and move is on the way. It's already starting to happen. I can see it in Somerville and other community programs. I can also see signs of it at scientific meetings across the country, in the legislative halls of Washington, D.C., in articles in the media, and in conversations with StrongWomen Program leaders across the country, with business leaders concerned about employee health and their bottom line, and with companies concerned with the greater population's well-being. The epidemic of inactivity, poor nutrition, and obesity is high on the national agenda. We have the knowledge and we have the emergence of political will.

In short, many of the elements of successful social change are now in place. We have a clearly defined crisis, backed by a large scientific base of information on the issue. We understand that there are substantial economic costs related to the problem; estimates put the price tag of the obesity epidemic at $270 billion a year in health-care costs alone. Perhaps more important, we also understand the human cost, especially to young people. Roughly a third of our children can expect to develop type 2 diabetes in their lifetime. Experts suggest that today's children will have a shorter lifespan than their parents. Until we reverse this epidemic, the population at large will continue to experience more elevated heart disease, arthritis, and several types of cancer, especially breast and colon cancers.

Many high-profile "spark plugs" have come forward, the best known being First Lady Michelle Obama. Numerous coalitions such as Neelam's and Barbara's have formed. There is abundant advocacy from a variety of groups, ranging from the NFL's "Fuel up to Play 60" to Sesame Street's "Healthy Habits for Life." The media is slowly showing more interest (witness Jamie Oliver's food revolution)—although we need more engagement here, and we need it now. Environmental shifts are beginning. Local, state, and national policies are changing, as evidenced by the reauthorization of the Child Nutrition Act (which includes significant changes to school lunches) and the development of large-scale plans such as the National Physical Activity Plan and a number of national obesity prevention plans.

People everywhere are waking up and realizing that their environment does not support healthy behaviors, and they are caring enough to create change. This is critical. We need more people acting now—especially women. Fortunately, more and more women are getting involved. This is the good news—that millions of women are reaching the conclusion that they want to make change in some facet of their own lives and to help create change in the lives of others.

We now know the power of social networks. Small and large, face-to-face and digital, these networks are critical to creating the change we need. Our challenge now is to motivate women across the country, to create a network of champions, to help women transform themselves, and thus empowered, become agents of change for their families, communities, and beyond. That is the goal of this book.

It's important that we not be too cautious in our individual and collective aspirations. Women sometimes worry too much about rocking the boat or upsetting the status quo. We don't like to be uncomfortable in social situations. We are going to have to break these patterns, to be bold and assertive. Our friends and family, our community, and most important, the next generation, deserve our best effort.

In May 2011, Ronit Ridberg, a graduate of the Friedman School of Nutrition Science and Policy at Tufts University, said it well when she addressed her fellow graduates in a commencement speech:

"In the old days, here's what used to happen: People would take food out of the ground and put it into their mouths. That's it. And that was called 'eating.' But something happened between the old days and today. A lot of things happened, in fact. Whole systems—economic, political, climatic, social, and agricultural systems—conspired against getting fresh food from the ground to people's mouths. To my fellow graduates, I say, 'Okay. It's time to change the world. No, seriously, it's time. We're actually going to have to do this."

We are at a unique moment in this country. Given how much is at stake and the scope of the challenges facing us, it's clear that we can't depend on others to take the necessary actions. It will take more than government and other institutional programs. It will take *us*, women helping ourselves, helping other people—one by one, community by community —until meaningful change goes viral throughout this country and we create an environment that promotes health for all.

I'm optimistic: I know we can do it.

Resources

I also maintain three online resources:

Website: strongwomen.com

Facebook site: Facebook.com/StrongWomenwithMiriam-Nelson

The interactive social media site for this book can be found at: SocialNetworkDiet.com

For information on my work at the John Hancock Research Center on Physical Activity, Nutrition, and Obesity Prevention at Tufts University's Friedman School of Nutrition, please go to our website: jhrc.nutrition.tufts.edu.

Websites of our Game Changers:

Neelam Sharma

Community Services Unlimited, Inc. (csuinc.org)

Barbara McCann

Complete Streets (completestreets.org)

Carla Marcus

WinterKids (winterkids.org)

Jill Vialet

Playworks, Inc. (playworks.org)

Online social networking sites related to health discussed in this book:

stickk.com

loseit.com

sparkpeople.com

Books of interest:

Christakis, Nicholas A. and James A. Fowler. *Connected: The Surprising Power of Our Social Networks and How They Shape Our Lives.* Little, Brown and Company, 2009.

Hesterman, Oran B. *Fair Food: Growing a Healthy, Sustainable Food System for All.* Public Affairs, 2011.

Kessler, David. *The End of Overeating: Taking Control of the Insatiable American Appetite.* Rodale, 2009.

Kirkpatrick, David. *The Facebook Effect: The Inside Story of the Company That Is Connecting the World.* Simon and Schuster, 2010.

Nestle, Marion. *Food Politics: How the Food Industry Influences Nutrition and Health.* University of California Press, 2007.

Pollan, Michael. *The Omnivore's Dilemma: A Natural History of Four Meals.* Penguin, 2007.

Sagawa, Shirley and Deborah Jospin. *The Charismatic Organization: 8 Ways to Grow a Nonprofit.* Jossey-Bass, 2008.

Tisch, Jonathan with Karl Weber. *Citizen You! Doing Your Part to Change the World.* Crown, 2010.

Wansink, Brian. *Mindless Eating: Why We Eat More Than We Think.* Bantam, 2006.

Government Resources:

Office on Women's Health

Department of Health and Human Services
200 Independence Avenue, SW, Room 712E
Washington, DC 20201
Telephone: 800-994-9662
Womenshealth.gov
Girlshealth.gov

Acknowledgments

Jennifer and I are deeply grateful for the generous support of the many people who assisted us in writing this book.

First and foremost, heartfelt thanks to Pamela Omidyar for believing in this project from the start and for providing essential funding for the research and writing of the book.

Tufts University has provided me with an environment that encourages innovative approaches to tackling major societal problems. A large network of Tufts colleagues contributed to the book. I want to thank all of my colleagues at the John Hancock Research Center on Physical Activity, Nutrition, and Obesity Prevention, especially Drs. Christina Economos, Sara Folta, Jennifer Sacheck, and Mr. Mark Fenton. My experience with our national StrongWomen initiative infused the entire book. Dr. Rebecca Seguin, Ms. Eleanor Heidkamp-Young, and thousands of StrongWomen leaders across the country deserve abundant thanks for their commitment to improving the health of women nationwide. Several graduate students provided invaluable assistance at various points during the writing, namely, Emily Kuross Vikre, Biz Morris Haselwandter, Bryan Stroup, and Allison Knott. Dr. Timothy Griffin at the Friedman School of Nutrition Science and Policy at Tufts University generously offered feedback on food policy. The end of the book would not be as strong without the powerful words of Ronit Ridberg. My colleagues Rob Hollister, Nancy Wilson, and Peter Levine, all at the Jonathan M. Tisch College of Citizenship and Public Service, were kind enough to provide me with their views on citizenship, public service, and social change. Thank you also to Jonathan Tisch for talking with me about his insight into citizenship and public service. Jennifer is deeply grateful to the Tisch College for her appointment as a Senior Fellow during the writing of this book. The Tufts President's Marathon Challenge team, especially President Lawrence Bacow, Eric Johnson, and Donald Megerle, showed me day in and day out the broad, positive reach that a strong social network can have on improving the health of thousands. Finally, a thank you to Peter Dolan, Jo Wellins, Cindy Briggs Tobin, and Jacqueline Kral for their continued guidance and support of my work.

Outside of Tufts University, Patricia Britten, MS, PhD, at the U.S. Department of Agriculture, Center for Nutrition Policy Promotion was a key source for information related to dietary intake of Americans.

Personal stories are essential to bringing concepts to light. I am indebted to Deanne Hobba and Martha Peterson for telling us their respective life stories—I am in awe of them both. Carla Marcus, Barbara McCann, Neelam Sharma, Jill Vialet, and the other twelve women who agreed to participate in our StrongWomen Move Mountains research project provided invaluable insight into the essential elements of creating meaningful social change. These women are all game changers.

During the writing of this book, Jennifer and I spent time together on several writing retreats. Dan O'Neill was kind enough to provide us with a lovely house on Elbow Mountain in Virginia. Dorrit Green and Michael Rodemeyer invited us to stay in their warm home in Charlottesville while they were away. We thank Tom and Ruth Earle and the Earle Family

Farm for nourishing us so well during one summer week up in New Hampshire.

Fran Newton, Ginger Barber, Holly Mauro, and Tim Galligan read early drafts of the manuscript and provided on-target comments that helped to shape the final book.

Our literary agents, Wendy Weil and Melanie Jackson, couldn't have been more supportive. We thank them both for all their guidance. All of our colleagues at FastPencil deserve special thanks, as they have been so enthusiastic about this project. Steve Wilson and Bruce Butterfield saw the scope and potential impact of building social networks for public good. Their enthusiasm has been infectious.

More so than ever before, our families contributed significantly to this book. Our husbands, Kin Earle and Karl Ackerman, offered support and wise advice throughout the project. And our children, Mason, Eliza, and Alexandra Earle and Zoë and Nell Ackerman, participated in and provided insight into many discussions around social networks, added sugars, food environment, walkable communities, etc. Some of them even read and provided feedback on various chapters. We love being at the center of their network.

Index

About the Authors

Miriam E. Nelson, Ph.D.

Miriam E. Nelson, Ph.D. is director of the John Hancock Research Center on Physical Activity, Nutrition, and Obesity Prevention and professor of Nutrition at the Friedman School of Nutrition Science and Policy at Tufts University. She is also a fellow of the American College of Sports Medicine. For the past 19 years, Dr. Nelson has been principal investigator of studies on exercise and nutrition, work supported by grants from the government and private foundations. From 2007 to 2008, Dr. Nelson served as the vice chair of the Physical Activity Guidelines Advisory Committee, whose report was used to develop the 2008 Physical Activity Guidelines for Americans for the U.S. Department of Health and Human Services. Most recently, she served on the 2010 Dietary Guidelines Advisory Committee for the U.S. Department of Agriculture and Health and Human Services.

Dr. Nelson is the founder and director of the StrongWomen Initiative, a community nutrition and physical activity program for midlife and older women. Forty states currently run this not-for-profit program. She has helped people learn how to stay younger, healthier, and stronger, and her research has revolutionized how people understand nutrition, strength training, aging, and health.

Dr. Nelson is the author of the international best-selling *Strong Women* book series. These nine titles, published in 14 languages, have sold more than a million copies worldwide. *Strong Women, Strong Bones* received the esteemed Books for a Better Life Award from the Multiple Sclerosis Society for best wellness book of 2000.

Dr. Nelson has appeared in her own PBS special entitled *Strong Women Live Well.* She has also been featured on other television and radio shows, including *The Oprah Winfrey Show, The Today Show, Good Morning America, ABC Nightly News,* CNN, NPR's *Fresh Air,* and the Discovery Channel.

Visit her website at www.strongwomen.com

The interactive social media site for this book can be found at: www.SocialNetworkDiet.com

Jennifer Ackerman

Jennifer Ackerman's most recent book is *Ah-Choo! The Uncommon Life of Your Common Cold* (Twelve, 2010). Her previous books include *Sex Sleep Eat Drink Dream: A Day in the Life of Your Body,* which has been published in twelve languages; *Chance in the House of Fate: A Natural History of Heredity;* and *Notes from the Shore.* She is also the co-author with Miriam Nelson of a book on women's health, *Strong Women's Guide to Total Health* (Rodale, 2010). A contributor to *The New York Times, National Geographic, Scientific American* and many other publications, she is the recipient of numerous awards and fellowships, including a 2004 NEA Literature Fellowship in Nonfiction and a grant from the Alfred P. Sloan Foundation. Her articles and essays have been included in several anthologies, among them *The Penguin Book of the Ocean* (2010), *Best American Science Writing* (2005), *The Nature Reader* (1996) and *Best Nature Writing* (1996). From 2007 to 2010, Ackerman was a Senior Fellow at the Tisch College of Citizenship and Public Service at Tufts University.

Visit her website at www.jenniferackerman.net

Published by FastPencil
http://www.fastpencil.com